MW01659695

The Hand Book:
An Informational Guide for Parents of Children With Hand Differences

NINA LIGHTDALE-MIRIC, MD & SARAH TUBERTY, OTD, OTR/L

Made Possible by the
American Foundation for Surgery of the Hand

ASSH
American Society for Surgery of the Hand

AFSH
American Foundation for Surgery of the Hand

822 West Washington Boulevard
Chicago, IL 60607

Published by American Society for Surgery of the Hand.

ISBN-10: 1-935121-55-3
ISBN-13: 978-1-935121-55-8
Library of Congress Control Number: 2022931132

Last digit is the print number: 10 9 8 7 6 5 4 3 2 1

Development Editors: Nina Lightdale-Miric, MD and Sarah Tuberty, OTD, OTR/L
Executive Vice President and CEO: Mark C. Anderson, FASAE, CAE
Publishing Director: Olivia Williams
Cover Design: Jennifer Hanasz
Compositor: Mindmax Technologies

To all children with hand differences, may you grow up empowered to follow your dreams.

To our parents, Reina and Charles, Katheryn and Dennis, who supported and loved us as we followed ours.

Foreword

The authors, Nina Lightdale-Miric and Sarah Tuberty, have done something very special and relevant in putting this book together. Based on their dedicated work as a pediatric hand surgeon and an occupational therapist who has a hand difference, they have given you, the family of the child with a limb difference, the accumulated wisdom of many years of caring for children like yours. This book will help you navigate the medical care information, emotions, and care options ahead as you embrace your new baby.

We have a combined experience of more than 60 years of caring for children with limb differences and their families at Texas Scottish Rite Hospital in Dallas and Shriners Children's Hospital in Sacramento. We have seen the triumphs and turmoil of our families and learned from them the joys and challenges that come with parenting children with limb differences. We are privileged to have been welcomed into many families and known many newborns into adulthood.

We know that once you recover from the shock of facing a future that is different from what you had imagined, you will see an amazing new human being eager for love, encouragement, and help in growing into a capable young person. We have learned that one of the most important things you can do for your child is to give him words for his entire world — and that includes words for his hand differences. Telling your child her own personal story will help her make sense of everything in her universe. Over these decades of our own work, we've seen the culture around children with physical differences shift toward more inclusion and empowerment.

Your child may not have two typical hands, yet he or she is still very much whole and complete. You have an amazing, growing child in your midst. Be awed!

Marybeth Ezaki, MD
Texas Scottish Rite Hospital

Michelle James, MD
Shriners Hospital for Children–Northern California

Preface

In this *Hand Book* you will find a guide, a starting point, an overview of the science, and a collection of information and resources from experts. You are offered discussion questions to help you sort through your feelings and guide the medical decisions you are making on behalf of your child throughout childhood.

Parents of a child with a hand difference share some of the same experiences of all parents, *plus* some unique challenges, feelings, and thoughts. Everyone's journey *is* different and if someone tells you that "everybody goes through this," remember that there's no rule or law that says you or your child must be an "everybody." *The Hand Book* is meant to help parents through every step of that process, from getting the "hand news" to watching your child leave for college.

This *Hand Book* is a neon WE ARE OPEN sign to a welcoming, safe, and knowledgeable medical place. We will explain terms, define conditions, introduce the range of treatments your health care team may recommend, discuss emotions, and offer coping techniques. Most importantly, we hope this book will help you feel confident that your child will grow up to be happy, empowered, and unlimited.

Nina Lightdale-Miric, MD
Sarah Tuberty, OTD, OTR/L

Contents

Foreword .... **iv**

Preface .... **v**

Part I: The Tools

Chapter 1
The Hand Guide: Setting Up 3

Chapter 2
The Hand News: Welcoming a New Family Member 17

Chapter 3
Hand Questions: Understanding What Causes Hand Differences (and What Doesn't) 25

Chapter 4
Hand Talk: Shaping Language to Shape Your World 39

Part II: Health Care

Chapter 5
Getting the Most out of Doctor Appointments and Opinions 51

Chapter 6
Hand Surgery: Indications and Techniques 61

Chapter 7
Hand Prosthesis: Exploring Tools 75

Chapter 8
Hand Therapy: Adaptations and Functional Training 85

Part III: Growing Up

Chapter 9
Stigma: Disability and Hand Differences 93

Chapter 10
A Support System: Cultivating Relationships with Friends and Family 107

Chapter 11
Branching Out: Finding Community 117

Chapter 12
Adapting Advocacy: Navigating School and the Government 127

Chapter 13
Creating Your Own Hand Book 137

Acknowledgments 139

About the Authors 143

References 147

Part I
The Tools

Chapter 1

The Hand Guide: Setting Up

In this Chapter

IN THIS CHAPTER, WE WILL LEARN:

- How this book works to help parents prepare and embrace the journey ahead
- How to use the references, discussion questions, and resources in this book to guide medical decisions in the care of a child with a hand difference

Welcome to *The Hand Book*! We are delighted and excited for you. This book is developed as an informational guide with discussion questions for each reader to consider independently. It is designed to be read and referenced in short sections at a time. Pick it up, flip to the section you are interested in, and then put it back down. There is a lot of content here. Use it as you need it, when you need it.

The Hand Book is the combination of the real-life experiences of its authors and the science known to date. Both authors have careers in serving families with congenital limb differences. The topics covered in this text are a collection of medical and psychosocial research, common-theme conversations we have had, and stories we have collected from parents and people with limb differences over the past 20 years. This is by no means an end-all-be-all; there is a lot of information in this book, and a lot of information that is not. We felt it was best to include topics that parents generally ask about. Please use this as a reference to begin your own research and to help guide the questions you may need to ask yourself or others. Welcome to this journey. We are so happy to have you with us.

Parents of a child with a hand difference will find their own pathways toward ensuring a happy and productive future for their child. Children with hand differences will find their own way too! Along this journey, there will be joys and surprises, and a few unknowns. Ultimately, with love as your guide, both you and your child will become knowledgeable and confident together.

Certain challenging experiences of raising a child with a hand difference are common and even predictable: birth announcements, making friends, starting school, medical decisions to make for your child, and, later, supporting your child's own choices. Most of those moments make your child's life a journey shared with all parents. The order and intensity of the stops or steps on the journey may be different for everyone involved. This is OK.

As a parent, the early stages of the journey may be a bit tricky. Navigating hospitals, surgeries, and therapists can make you feel that you are in a different world than other new parents. As a parent, it's important that you maintain your own physical and mental well-being in addition to tending to your child's and partner's needs. Life can quickly become complicated, so putting together a plan is important—especially when it comes to unexpected stops along the way. A solid plan framework will empower you when making decisions and prepare you to face obstacles when you meet them.

You and your child are going to be OK. In fact, you're both going to be better than OK. This experience may not be what you expected, nor what you planned for, yet your love and commitment to your child will rise above all else. The joys, magic, and challenges of raising a child with a hand difference are ahead!

In this first chapter we will talk about setting up the tools that allow you to work on caring for yourself, facing your fears, and making medical decisions, and briefly touch on finances. Keep referring back to this introductory chapter while reading through the following materials. Much of the content is for inspiration, and discussion questions are placed throughout to provoke thoughts and help guide your personalized decisions on this journey.

LET'S TALK LANGUAGE

The word "parent" is used in this book to identify anyone who takes on a parenting role for a child with a limb difference. Parents can be biological, step, adoptive, foster, relatives, or whoever is the guardian most committed to this child's health. The term "you" used throughout this text is in reference to anyone providing a parental role. Children are referred to as "they" within the text for inclusiveness.

This book will refer to "hand difference" or "limb difference" interchangeably. Some families prefer "hand difference," as this helps differentiate "upper limb" from "lower limb." This book uses both terminologies, and you can choose whatever words you feel work best for your child and your family. The term "congenital" refers to a limb difference that is present at birth. The term "acquired" means at birth a person had both hands, and then at some point along their life journey they obtained a limb difference. Although tools, strategies, and information could likely be transferred, the functional and psychosocial impacts of a congenital hand difference are different for those who acquired hand differences. This book is written with a focus on congenital hand differences.

The medical language and terminology used to describe this topic has varied and will continue to evolve over the years. "Hand differences" was chosen for this text as "hand" is inclusive of all variations of the upper limb, fingers, arm, and shoulder. If a child has a difference in their shoulder, there will be a difference in their hand. If their hand is absent, that is a hand difference. We acknowledge that the term "difference" may evolve in the future. Please feel empowered to use the terminology that resonates with you and your family.

This book will introduce themes on stigma, differences, and disability. The terms "different" and "disability" are both viewed positively and used positively in this text. While these terms are physical, cultural, or legal terms at heart, currently they drive a positive movement of advocacy, identity, and pride. Understanding what "disability" and "different" mean today may be a way to help support the positive identity development of your child's limb difference with your child, family, and community.

THE VERY FIRST STEP IS CARING FOR YOURSELF

Lots of parents have described their initial reactions when learning that their child has a hand difference. The reality is, it may not be the news you expected to hear, and there is an entire process that is associated with learning that your child has a limb difference. Parents have found that their own health is not looked after and they may feel isolated. Please know that you are not alone! This section will cover some positive coping strategies and the importance of taking care of yourself first, so you are prepared to take care of your new family.

Have you ever noticed the oxygen mask in the safety demonstration on an airplane? "In case of emergency, you should put on your own oxygen mask before you try to assist others." It's the same for parents of children with hand differences. Sometimes, it's easy to get caught up in taking care of everyone else and you forget to put on your own oxygen mask. *Care for yourself so you can care for your child.*

When some people hear *self-care,* they imagine a day off, exploring the outdoors, getting a massage, or eating amazing food. While that might be a great idea from time to time, the overall idea of wellness and self-care is much broader. Are you getting enough sleep? Are you eating enough fruits and vegetables? Or drinking enough water? Taking the time for a drive or walk or half hour to just be with your partner (or alone) can work wonders. Try a breathing exercise on an app on your phone, write in your journal, or listen to music. All these activities can make a bigger difference than you might expect for both your physical and mental health.

They provide you the space to take a step back and reflect on your experiences and set you up to take on the next step. You can find reflective time with loved ones, with a therapist, or in a support group.

It's important that multiple parents and caregivers adjust and balance their own mental and physical health with each other as well. Maybe your partner will have the same or different needs. Recognize the important space each of you may need to re-center when knocked off balance.

Do Regular Check-ins

Set milestones and check-ins for yourself. Fill out a status check each week or month and see how you're doing compared to the month prior. As you answer each question, look back at your past answers and see what has changed. Before you know it, you'll begin to feel more empowered and more in control. Create space to chat with your partner or a co-parent about their experience and do regular check-ins with them. You both may be experiencing similar things but at different times.

Keep track of your own behaviors and have others help you reflect on them. Maybe you are unconsciously exhibiting isolating behaviors such as covering up your child in the store or avoiding Parent and Me classes, the park, or preschool. Call yourself out when doing these things. Then, forgive yourself. It's normal to do it and can be healthy. There is a balance here. Full isolation is not a rewarding policy for interacting with the world all of the time. While you want to be engaged with the world, everyone needs a break sometimes. However, when you're avoiding more than engaging, maybe it's time to challenge yourself to get out a bit more.

Older children may enter periods when they just don't feel like talking about their hands. They'll pull down their sleeve, put their limb into their pocket, keep a tight group of friends, or stay away from new things or places. That's fine sometimes. When this avoidance gets in the way of joy and social engagement, then it's not fine. The more you practice finding the balance in yourself, the better you'll be able to teach your child to do the same. That idea of preparing yourself and child with coping techniques for expected challenges such as people staring or being discriminated against is often called packing a "crisis bag."

Create a Crisis Bag

Some people find creating a crisis bag helpful when feeling overwhelmed. Your "bag" (or box or drawer) can be a premade collection of items to help facilitate coping and the ability to center your emotions. Think of things that stimulate the senses, like a favorite fidget toy, picture, or scented object. Create a playlist of songs that ground or center you. Include something soft like a blanket or hard like a tactile bead. Perhaps include a journal and a nice pen. Your bag can include a collection of positive things like empowering quotes or nice things people have said about you or your child to help reframe your thoughts. When you feel yourself entering a crisis, pull out this bag and interact with the various items to help bring yourself back. Even taking the 20 minutes to reflect is beneficial.

Don't be afraid to reach out to people you trust who know you, support you, and care about you. If needed, reach out to health care professionals so they can assist with more tools to help keep you crisis-free.

Your well-being is critically important to successfully parenting your child. Parents of all types of children may feel guilty when they take time for themselves. This guilt can be worse if you're worried that your child with a limb difference may need you while you're not there. But remember, your own care is part of putting your oxygen mask on first. It's harder to assist others if you aren't caring for yourself first. You will do your best for your family when you are your best self. You become your best self when you take care of yourself.

CARING FOR YOURSELF WORKSHEET

Date:

Mental/Physical Check-In: On a scale of 1 to 10 (with 10 being highest),

HOW DO I FEEL TODAY?

Mental Health

1	2	3	4	5	6	7	8	9	10
☐	☐	☐	☐	☐	☐	☐	☐	☐	☐

Physical Health

1	2	3	4	5	6	7	8	9	10
☐	☐	☐	☐	☐	☐	☐	☐	☐	☐

1. **What did I do for my mental health today/this week?**
2. **What did I do for my physical health today/this week?**
3. **What would I like to change?**
4. **What are 3 helpful things that make me feel better when I am upset?**

FACING YOUR FEARS IS PART OF SELF-CARE

A big step in coping will be facing your personal "fear of the unknown" for your child with a hand difference. Sometimes the source of this fear will seem obvious, like bullying or an upcoming surgery. Other times, fear may be more unplanned, like an unexpected emotional response in the supermarket. Your fear may be generated by your own childhood, your culture, your family environment, or events of the day. You may feel like you are the only one accountable for everything from insurance and finances to the potential bullies on your child's playground.

Discussing these fears openly helps you face them. By talking about them with a partner, a family member, a close friend, or your therapist, or even writing them down in a journal, you'll feel better prepared to tackle fears head-on. Once you've identified those fears of the unknown you can create a plan for facing them. Saying them out loud will prepare you for strong emotions you may feel when they are triggered along the way.

Your worry may be a "micro-worry," such as an upcoming doctor appointment, or a "macro-worry," such as wondering if your child will have friends, play happily, get a driver's license, or get married someday. All these thoughts and concerns are legitimate and valid. Make a note on when small things are feeling big. Remember, fears of the unknown are not reality.

Parents have dreams for their children and hope they have good jobs, fall in love, and live successful, long, and meaningful lives. Parents may have general fears that their child will experience pain, hurt, failure, bullying, or harm. Their instincts to fiercely protect their child from emotional injury or social isolation can even generate anger. The more you own those fears, the better you can identify situations that trigger fear or protective behavior in you. This enables you to choose how you want to respond in these situations instead of simply reacting.

As you work through many of your worries, you'll find that your child will create their own resiliency, influenced by behavior you model for them as a parent. By organizing your thoughts and addressing your own fears in a healthy way, you give your child tools in their own coping toolbox. Instead of a hammer, screwdriver, and wrench, your child will learn from you when and how to use their words and actions to build their world and keep themselves safe even when you are not there.

Dr Eileen Bradbury, a prominent research psychologist in children with physical differences, is quoted as saying, "Children can learn to live with anything if they believe they are loved and lovable." Teach your children how to love and be loved in return. Some adults who have hand differences have come to see themselves with a gift that allows them a unique journey through this world, achieving fulfillment and happiness in ways others without differences might miss out on.

FACING YOUR FEAR WORKSHEET

Date:

On a scale of 1 to 10 (with 10 being highest),

HOW FEARFUL OF THE UNKNOWN SURROUNDING MY CHILD AM I TODAY?

1	2	3	4	5	6	7	8	9	10
☐	☐	☐	☐	☐	☐	☐	☐	☐	☐

1. **What am I most afraid of in raising my child with a hand difference? How realistic or likely to happen is that feared experience or event?**
2. **What am I joyful and excited about when raising my child with a hand difference?**
3. **What 3 steps will I take (or continue taking) to address my fears and concerns?**

MAKING MEDICAL DECISIONS

As you work through this book and consider various medical decisions on behalf of your child, you will be attempting to incorporate your child's future wants and needs. Perhaps you can clearly see areas where your child could benefit from medical care and areas where they are doing just fine without intervention. We encourage you to consider all opportunities while making medical care decisions. Discuss options with your family, medical care team, and those who are involved in the health and development of your child. When they are older, share with your child the options they have at a level that is developmentally appropriate for them and allow them the space to provide feedback. Research has shown that neurotypically developing children around 8 years old have the awareness to make sound medical decisions when explained at a level they understand. Find out which medical decisions are time dependent and may need to be completed while the child is young, as the results might not be as effective.

Medical decisions on behalf of children who cannot participate, like many other areas of parenting, are not always clear and easy. They may come with thoughts such as "I'm pretty sure," and "It's just what I feel is right to me," and "What if I'm wrong?" Writing down your thoughts and influences around the decisions now will help you explain them to yourself and your child later.

It's important when making these decisions (and legally required when you sign consent for surgery) that you feel you have enough information to make the decision. Take the time to ask questions of those who should know the answers. If you need more information, you can speak to other experts, involve a larger care team, ask for another appointment, speak on the phone, or send an email to the health care professionals with follow-up questions. You may benefit from meeting other parents who've chosen a particular surgery or treatment for their child, too.

Some parents may feel pressure from family or friends to make certain medical decisions before they are ready. Create a healthy environment around you when making such decisions. This will allow you to clearly see each influence on that decision. It's beneficial to reflect on your own reactions and their source. If you have a strong reaction to a possible treatment option, such as a surgery to straighten a child's wrist or move a toe to their hand, where does that come from? Is it fear of the unknown? Is it fear that your child would or would not have wanted you to make that decision on their behalf? Or is it something else? Recognizing your triggers and the source of your worry is important. Do what you need to feel empowered to make your own educated and thoughtful decisions for the care of your child.

Use the information and science from your medical team, your community, and within this book to guide your personalized medical decisions. The following worksheet can help you organize information as you learn it. You are not expected to complete this worksheet now. Use it as you learn more about options.

MEDICAL DECISIONS WORKSHEET

1. What is my child's limb difference? Identify the medical term, diagnosis, or general description of the limb difference.
2. What are my child's strengths when using their arms? List both creative/problem-solving skills and the physical strengths they have.
3. What barriers or challenges are they facing?
4. What are my potential options, and what are the goals of each option?
5. Are any of the options time sensitive and needing decisions by a certain date?
6. What research (speaking with other parents or adult children who have had these interventions, research articles, second opinions) can be found for each of the options?
7. Do any of the interventions conflict with each other? Can they be done synchronously?
8. What are the downsides of each option? Consider cost, time off work, etc.
9. What are people telling me that I should do? And do I want to do that?
10. What do I want?
11. What does my child want, or what do I think my child would want? Be sure to talk about it in a way that matches their developmental understanding.
12. What does my partner or co-parent want?
13. After reviewing all the pieces, what do we value as a family?
14. What decision will we as a family make? Making a decision to not make a decision at this time is both a decision in itself and an option here. Set a date or a milestone to revisit medical decisions and determine if you want to make a different decision at that time.

Once you've made a decision, consider how you will communicate your family's decision to those around you. Know that their opinions and reactions are not a reflection of you or your decision-making skills. You can share with family members that you made a decision and ask them to support you in it.

Consider how you want to communicate your decisions to your children as they grow older. You can very personally write your child a letter (or record a video) while you are in the space of making the decisions. You can give them this letter or video, or whatever media form you like most for your child, when they are older—say, 8 or 13 years old—as a way to help communicate to them why you made the choices you did when they were younger.

SETTING UP FINANCES

A new baby changes your personal finances. Along this journey, having a child with a hand difference may include some unexpected costs. Money, time from work, and health insurance coverage may be obstacles to obtaining some of the medical care and creating the ideal, supportive environment for your child. You may (or may not) have excellent health insurance, but it still may not cover all your expenses, especially travel to see medical specialists, therapists, and prosthetists. Once your child has been evaluated and you have decided on a treatment path, your doctor's office/clinic/hospital can assist you with financial options.

Certain hospital systems, summer camps, or other programs and events may be philanthropically funded and relatively low cost or even cost-free for your child's health care needs. These institutions may be further from your home; therefore, there may be more hidden costs such as transportation, hotels, and food.

After reviewing all these options, create a financial plan that works for your child and for your family. Determine the best ways to save, identify sponsorship/scholarships, and identify support from your community to help you and your family.

Much of this step is routine for most parents, as having a child always involves some financial planning. However, educating yourself about financial needs that may be unique to this child, then tackling them head-on, will help you as you make your own personal plan.

FINANCES WORKSHEET

Financial Check-In: On a scale of 1 to 10 (with 10 being highest),

HOW COMFORTABLE AM I WITH OUR FAMILY'S FINANCES?

1	2	3	4	5	6	7	8	9	10
☐	☐	☐	☐	☐	☐	☐	☐	☐	☐

1. **How do my child's care needs change what I planned for while I was pregnant?**
2. **What does my financial landscape look like? Identify assets (saving accounts, retirement accounts, invested funds).**
3. **Identify financial needs you have currently and ones that will be coming soon (out-of-pocket medical, therapy, and/or prosthetic costs, etc.). Include large purchases such as home repairs or additional car payments.**
4. **What are financial areas that are unplanned or unexpected?**
5. **Where can I secure funds (even if it is a collection of multiple sources)? Examples are insurance coverage, scholarships, past savings that can cover costs, and family support.**
6. **Write out your budget. Is there a way to reprioritize needs to ensure that my family can cover necessary costs? Will I be able to ensure financial stability for the whole family?**

CHAPTER SUMMARY

In this chapter, we learned:

- How to use this *Hand Book* to empower yourself in raising a child with a hand difference
- Ways to think through your own health, fears, medical decision making, and finances
- To enjoy the journey. Whether you have just given birth or whether your child has just gone to college, you should remember to take the time to savor and enjoy the wild, wonderful ride of parenting your child.

Chapter 2

The Hand News: Welcoming a New Family Member

In this Chapter

IN THIS CHAPTER, WE WILL LEARN:

- Ways of processing your unique "hand news" emotions
- Ways to define a baseline for your child and yourself
- Ways of navigating the hospital after giving birth
- How to explore choosing the best language for your new family

THE HAND NEWS

Here is the hand news: your child was born with a hand difference. Breathe. This is more than news—it is a journey with a full and meaningful life. How it begins may be crucial to how events evolve.

The first time you hear the hand news is the day you discover that your child has a hand difference. Perhaps it was on an ultrasound image, in a photo from an adoption agency, or in the delivery room. Your doctors may use complicated or confusing terms like "congenital" or "anomaly." Feelings of fear and worry may overshadow your joy in becoming a parent. You have prepared for your baby for months or years, imagining your life with your new family member, and this was not part of your image of being a parent. Some parents describe feeling frozen, in shock, surrounded by silence, or watching the world move in slow motion at the first realization that their child has different arms, hands, or fingers than expected. For some parents, the hand news is a profound loss of the world they had imagined for their new child.

Some parents feel helpless that they can't protect their child from harm, fix it, or make the differences go away. Many, many parents blame themselves, asking, "What did I do wrong?" Other parents or relatives who have inherited hand differences ("it runs in the family") feel responsible for having passed this on to their new child. For them, thoughts are influenced by their own experience and journey through life with a hand difference.

DISCUSSION QUESTIONS

Most people form memories with emotions, and likely feel more than one at once.

What are some of the emotions you felt when you heard the hand news?

Have they changed today? If so, what are some of the changes?

When you feel the earth is back on its axis, you can reopen your mind to a new definition of normal. You are not the first parents to do this. Your child is not the only child out there with a hand difference. Though your feelings may be complex or confusing, they are very real, so give yourself permission to experience them. Based on the feelings parents have shared with us over the years, and based on comments from researchers in published papers, parents of children with limb differences have some common emotions. Parents can feel all of these emotions at the same time, which can feel confusing. Take time to learn more about them and reflect on the emotions you are experiencing.

Joy: Parents can feel joy for bringing a child into the world, joy for the celebration of this new human, and excitement for the life they will lead. Joy is defined by Brené Brown in her research as "an intense feeling of deep spiritual connection, pleasure, and appreciation." Joy can also be a very vulnerable feeling.

Love: A combination of joy and trust, love is what parents feel for their child. This love facilitates bonding, attachment, and commitment to their child, and the child often mirrors this back to the parents.

Grief: A more intense feeling of sadness associated with a loss. Parents may feel mournful over the loss of the child they expected and feel intense sadness when imagining what the future may hold for their child. Brown discussed research from Tashel Bordere on "disenfranchised grief," which is defined as grief that "is not openly acknowledged or publicly supported through mourning practices or rituals because the experience is not valued or counted."

Guilt: Defined by Brown as "an emotion we experience when we fall short of our own expectations or standards." The focus is on the action done. Parents may feel guilty that they brought a child with something different into the world.

Shame: Defined by Brown as "the intensely painful feeling or experience of believing that we are flawed and therefore unworthy of love, belonging, and connection." Shame focuses on the self versus the action, and according to Brown's research, shame needs judgment, secrecy, and silence to flourish. Many parents may feel that they are flawed by bringing to life a child who has a difference.

Anger: Parents may feel angry. Some feel angry that they have to bear this burden while they look at other perfect-seeming children of their friends and family. Other parents may begin to blame this difference on the child or their partner. Anger can be a displaced emotion. It may be that parents are feeling other emotions and are unable to articulate and express them, so it may come out as anger.

Fear and anxiety: Parents may feel afraid of raising a child with a hand difference or fear for the difficulties their child will experience. They may also have anxieties related to the overall health of their child and their child's ability to live a full and meaningful life. Cultural expectations can greatly increase this anxiety.

This is not an all-inclusive list of every emotion that you may have. Not everyone feels things the same way. However, it's important to remember that you are not alone in experiencing these emotions, even the uncomfortable ones. Take time to learn more about them and reflect on the emotions you are experiencing. These types of more intense emotions may lead to isolation of individuals or families but may also be felt and shared to lead to deeper understanding. Some parents will begin to cope and learn how to regulate these emotions, perhaps by doing the regular check-ins as described in Chapter 1. Other parents may benefit from more support in this area and may find seeing a therapist or counselor helpful.

THE FIRST FEW STEPS FORWARD

If you've just given birth, your obstetrician, a pediatrician who is on call, and any number of nurses and medical assistants helping you recover will be busily entering and leaving your hospital room. Medical technicians may arrive for tests, and family members will want to see you and the new baby. There will be phone calls, social media posts, and maybe an offer from the hospital photographer. Every virtual and in-person "knock" on your door can seem confusing while you are attempting to process new and conflicting emotions, excited to get started with parenting, yet now worried for your new baby. If you are still pregnant when you get the hand news, then seeing specialists and undergoing testing may be ahead.

Emotions are complex. Your health care team most likely understands that you may be both joyful and worried for your new child. Remember that people around you are there to help. When you are mindful of your emotions, you'll gain an awareness that can help you work with your family, your friends, and members of your care team in a more effective way.

Remember that you and your partner are in control of who is in your virtual and real space and who is not. At your very own thoughtful healthy pace, introduce your child to others, post to social media, or return calls. You can ask friends and family to come back later, or you can have them stay and be part of the space—whichever feels right. You can tell them or not tell them about the hand news. After all, you might not fully understand what's happening yet. There are no rules for this. Let others know if you need help. Be you in that moment, be real, keep breathing, put one foot in front of the other. Get ready to move forward in baby steps, not leaps, in space and time around you.

BONDING WITH BABY

Bonding with your new baby is an important first step in being a new parent. Bonding helps your child feel secure and connected to rely on you as a parent to care for them. The parent's bonding develops a truly specialized emotional attachment between parent and baby. Some parents feel this bond when first seeing their child, and other parents develop this bond over time. Having a hand difference and navigating through layers of guilt or grief may slow down the bonding process. This is OK. Be as slow and patient as you need to be while taking active steps to facilitate this bond: talking and singing to your child, holding them, smiling at them, and observing them smiling back at you.

Seeing your child as whole and deserving of your love and support is the goal of bonding.

POSTPARTUM SCIENCE

If you've recently given birth, it's worth noting that there may be a significant factor outside your control influencing what you're feeling right now. Approximately 70% to 80% of all new parents report some surprising mood changes and even negative feelings, commonly referred to as the "baby blues." It is absolutely normal to feel a range of emotions when having a new child due to a change in sleep patterns as well as a large number of hormones creating physical and chemical changes. There are significant ups and downs which can sometimes shift from minute to minute. It is important to be mindful of how these emotions are impacting your daily life.

New mothers and fathers who don't hear enough about postpartum depression often feel alone. Having a baby "should be" a joyous event. In that joy, however, your sleep patterns are disrupted. You now have a feeding schedule dictated by your new child. Often, your own needs are met last, if met at all. If you have just given birth, your body has completely changed. Your relationship with your partner, family, friends, and work might be going through some stress as well. Life has changed and many new parents find it hard to sort out these new and complex emotions from what may be signs of oncoming postpartum depression. Add a child with any type of difference to the equation, and feelings can quickly stack on top of each other.

DISCUSSION QUESTIONS

Reflect on the early days after your baby arrived.

What things, if any, have changed?

Is this your first child?

If not, what were your emotions after your other children were born?

Are they the same or different from what you are experiencing now? Distinguishing which emotions are related to being a new parent versus those emotions associated with having a child with a hand difference may help.

Perinatal depression is defined by the National Institute of Mental Health as a "mood disorder that affects women during pregnancy and after childbirth. Mothers experience extreme sadness, anxiety and fatigue that make it difficult for them to care for themselves or others."

Postpartum depression includes self-blame—feelings like anxiety, fear, worry, and panic without a good reason—and sometimes a risk of harm for the parent or child.

It's natural for parents to struggle with these new emotions and even feel shame when they can't always exude joy and happiness, as they think this is what society expects of them. You're not a bad parent by feeling these things, merely a very real parent. Keep talking about your feelings and share with your medical team if you need more support.

Find people who you trust, like your spouse, family members, parents, and friends. Identify people to support you as you share these emotions within a shame-free environment. Talk with your health care team. Ask about resources to help you understand your emotions and develop ways to manage them.

DISCUSSION QUESTIONS

1. Remember, no 2 people will experience their feelings about having a child with a congenital hand difference in the same way. Each child will travel their own path (although your role in guiding your child is crucial). Remember why you wanted to be a parent in the first place? Write or record a few lines about how you felt when you knew you would become a parent…Breathe!
2. What information are you receiving from the medical team? What needs does your baby have? What needs do you have? How can you best address them? Write down everything you can remember of what your doctors have said. Then write or record what you need at the moment. Don't worry about what you'll need tomorrow or next week. Be here now and just…Breathe!
3. Reflect on hearing the hand news and meeting your new child:
    a. What was your hand news day like?
    b. Do you remember how you felt?
    c. What do you feel that you needed at that moment?
    d. What are some happy memories of that day?
    e. What questions are you glad you asked, and how have things changed since then?
    f. What are some special things you did to bond with your new baby?
    g. What are you looking forward to doing together as a family this week, or this year, or in the future?

CHAPTER SUMMARY

In this chapter, we learned that:

- Hand differences happen. They may be unexpected, and naturally parents have a lot of healthy feelings around them.
- You are in control of how and when to tell people and who is in your space.
- You, your child, and your family are all going to be OK. Breathe!

Chapter 3

Hand Questions: Understanding What Causes Hand Differences (and What Doesn't)

In this Chapter

IN THIS CHAPTER, WE WILL LEARN:

- How the human hand forms
- Why congenital hand differences may occur
- About the types of hand differences

"Was it something I did?" It's a question that every parent of a child with a hand difference may ask themselves. The informed, science-based answer is NO! Believing and accepting this is critical to moving forward. It will also be important for your child to understand much later.

So, then, how did your child's hand difference happen? And why? The answer is, to the best of all knowledge, for the most part, still unknown. Unknowns are definitely disappointing, but once you have a better understanding of how and why your child's difference formed, you'll know that it could not have been prevented. Also, by knowing how hand differences are formed, you and your child will be empowered to educate others.

WHO HAS HAND DIFFERENCES?

Children with hand differences are of all races, on all continents, and from all cultures. Statistics are only estimates. The United States Centers for Disease Control and Prevention (CDC), World Health Organization (WHO), and regional- and country-specific data collectors reported the following statistics at the time this book was written:

- 5 of every 10,000 newborns have some difference in the arm, hand, forearm, or fingers.
- Congenital absence of the entire limb or hand was reported to occur in 6 per 100,000 children. At current birth rates, that would approximate over 200 children born every year in the United States without fingers on 1 or more limbs.
- Of all the children born without fingers on the hand, according to recent data, approximately three quarters are male. The left side is involved in two-thirds of the cases, and only 1% have differences in both hands. Fewer than 10% were ever found to have a family history or an identified genetic link.
- Most children born with a hand difference are otherwise without any health issues at all. Only 1 out of 10 children with a hand difference have other differences elsewhere on or in their body.

HOW HANDS FORM

The science of how a single fertilized embryo cell grows into a full-term newborn baby over approximately 9 months (or 40 weeks) of gestation (pregnancy) is called embryology. Once the egg is fertilized, the embryo rapidly divides. In the first 4 weeks, the cells take the shape of a tube. Somites or segments stack up like blocks that will become unique parts of the body, and the brain tissue collects at the top with a spinal cord along the back. Then, the outpouching or branches of this tube first become the arms and then legs while the heart, kidneys, and digestive system are forming in the center from about 4 to 8 weeks. There are several models of limb growth and which one is correct is still being studied. There are 3 defined segments: shoulder, elbow, and hand. There are also 2 sides: the back and the palm. Finally, there are 3 unique columns of growth: the thumb, the middle, and the pinky. The bones, joints, nerves, tendons, nails, and muscles slowly fill in and take shape. At 7 to 8 weeks, the initially webbed fingers separate into individual digits and the form of the entire limb is complete. For the remaining 28 weeks or so, the limbs grow mostly only in size. The entire process is truly amazing!

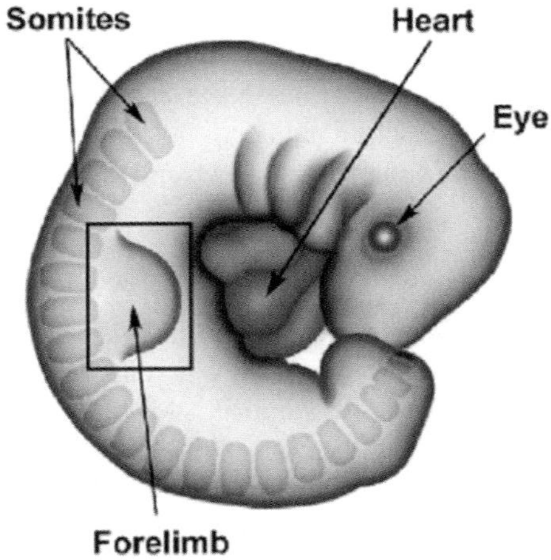

Figure 3-1: A human embryo at 4 weeks gestation (1 month pregnant) with upper limb bud starting. During this phase, intrinsic factors influence formation of the arm, hand, and fingers.

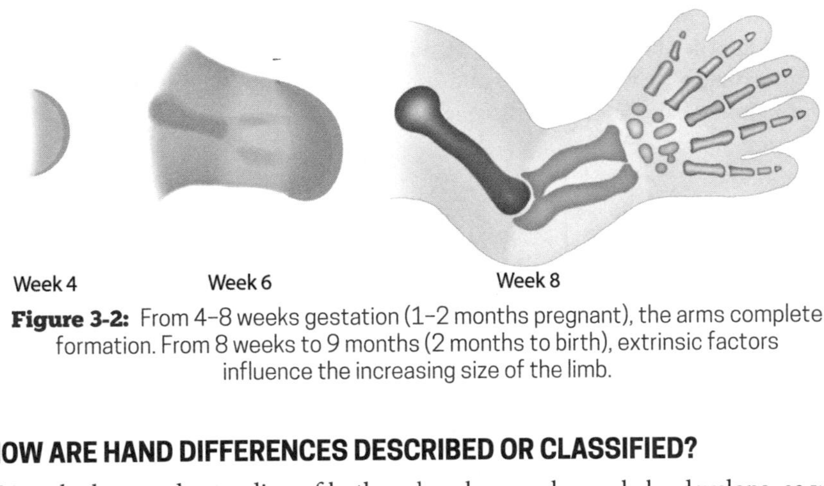

Figure 3-2: From 4–8 weeks gestation (1–2 months pregnant), the arms complete formation. From 8 weeks to 9 months (2 months to birth), extrinsic factors influence the increasing size of the limb.

HOW ARE HAND DIFFERENCES DESCRIBED OR CLASSIFIED?

Using the best understanding of both embryology, or how a baby develops, as well as molecular genetics, limb differences can be organized by the Oberg, Manske, and Tonkin (OMT) classification system into 4 types: *malformations*, *deformations*, *dysplasias*, and those caused by *genetic syndromes*. This classification system was adopted by the International Federation of Societies for Surgery of the Hand in 2014 and helps combine development and presentation of hand differences. This classification system is reviewed every 3 years for changes if needed. These terms are used in medical literature but may be different from what you find on the internet or the language your health care team uses if they do not have training in this field.

Malformations

Malformations of upper limb or hand formation are differences that formed from the very beginning. They come from those initial arm buds and occur before the eighth week of pregnancy and often before parents are aware they are pregnant. Examples of malformations include duplication (too many thumbs/fingers), over/undergrowth (limbs that are smaller or bigger), and congenital absence of the limb (it was never formed).

Some, but not all, of these sorts of differences start in the genes. To understand DNA or genes, think of it as instructions or blueprints for how the child's hand will be formed. The hand development may be as much of who they are and how they develop as their eye color or natural abilities. When the limb started to form but, for some reason we do not understand, stopped midway, bumps or "nubbins"—little round undeveloped fingers with fingernails—may be at the end of the limb or hand. Depending on when it stopped growing, the limb may form to the upper arm, elbow, wrist, or base of the fingers. This hand malformation is called symbrachydactyly or a transverse deficiency. If one of the columns or sides does not form, the hand will be without a thumb, middle part of the hand, or pinky finger. These are called longitudinal deficiencies and there are 3 types: radial, central, and ulnar. If the thumb side isn't there, it is called a radial longitudinal deficiency. If it is the pinky finger side, it is called an ulnar longitudinal deficiency. If it's the middle of the hand, it is called central deficiency (a split or cleft hand).

Other malformations of the hand include too many fingers (polydactyly) or even too many hands or arms (dimelia).

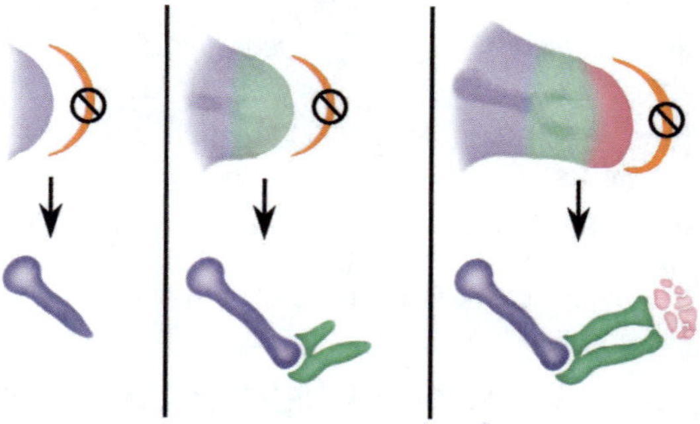

Figure 3-3: This is an example of research bringing science closer to discovering why a human child's limb might not form completely. The fingernails or endcap of the limb bud (in orange) seems to contain the messaging center that organizes the steps of forming each segment of the limb. In animal embryo studies, that area was removed at 3 different phases, and as a result, the shoulder (A), forearm (B), or hand (C) did not grow from that point on.

Deformations

Hand deformation is a result of an injury to an already developed limb. An example is the constriction rings (bands) around 3 to 4 months of pregnancy that may form from the amniotic sac. These rings of loose tissue can tighten around a finger or limb. The cause is unknown. Typically, these children have rings on more than 1 hand, swellings or puffiness in the hand, webbing mostly around the tips of the fingers, and no nubbins or fingernails on the affected digits. Doctors use these clues to distinguish deformations from malformations.

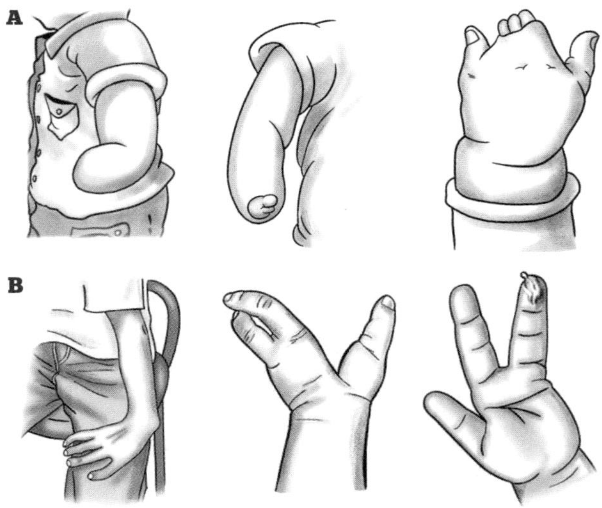

Figure 3-4 A and B: Malformations occur as intrinsic factors create a limb that is over or underdeveloped. Examples: (A) transverse deficiency, symbrachydactyly at the forearm, and symbrachydactyly at the hand/fingers. More examples: (B) radial longitudinal deficiency, cleft hand or central deficiency, and ulnar longitudinal deficiency.

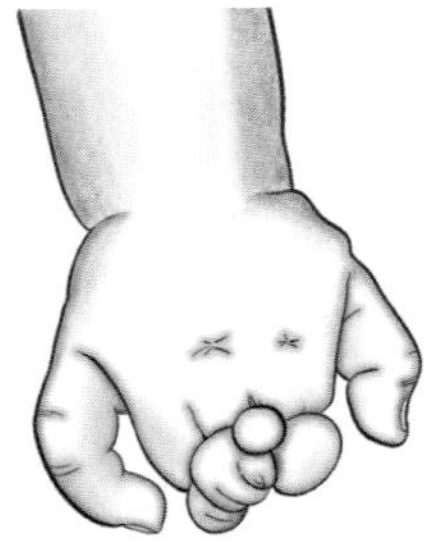

Figure 3-5: Deformations occur as extrinsic factors influence the growth of the limb, such as constriction bands, which wrap around the limb or fingers and cause deep creases, swelling, skin fusions, and amputations.

Dysplasias

Dysplasia is a way to describe unexpected growth ("dys" = abnormal + "plasia" = growth). Dysplastic growth can occur in any part of the body. Some may be caused by benign (not cancer) conditions that change the shape of the hand or limb. These growths can be small at first and increase in size along with the child to cause differences in hand shape and function over time.

Genetic Syndromes

Molecular genetics science, including researching the DNA from parents and children with limb differences, is becoming more advanced each year. Some syndromes are caused by a gene which can be passed through generations or appear for the first time in a baby when no other family members show the same condition. One example is TAR, or thrombocytopenia-absent radius syndrome, where the bones of both forearms are curved and shortened. Another example is the split hand/split foot gene that causes the central portion of both the hands and the feet to be cleft or small. Since some conditions are associated with problems in other organ systems, your child will likely have tests to check for that. As we discussed at the beginning of the chapter, 90% of children born without one arm or hand have no known genetic syndrome or other medical diagnosis. So, it's worth noting that hand differences that are part of genetic syndromes are even less common.

LEARNING MORE

Do you know the type of hand difference your child has? Once you give something a name, you can begin to learn about it. You may not know exactly why it happened, but writing its name down or saying it out loud can make it easier to research and learn about. Be mindful about any information you may find on the internet, and know that personal blogs are spaces where anyone with any background can comment or post information and call it "factual." Use the Check the Credibility Worksheet to assist you in evaluating information.

CHECK THE CREDIBILITY WORKSHEET

1. Who is the author? Is it a person, team of people, or an organization?
2. What are their credentials? More credible sources are people who have worked in the field for several years, have education and training in the topic presented, and have produced other works in similar areas.
3. Where is this information located? Is it in a blog post, a website, a magazine, a book, a research article? Think about the editing process with each location. Was there an opportunity for others who are trained in similar topics to provide feedback on the content written? Or was this a post made with little fact checking?
4. Are references included? References help support the information provided in the text to help ensure that it is based on research versus an individual idea. If references are listed, are they relevant to the same or similar topics as the content you are researching?
5. When was this information published? Information and research constantly evolve. Sources published within the past 10 years are more credible than work written before the past decade.
6. Ask your care team for sources of good, accurate, and up-to-date information.

Use this helpful checklist to determine if your source is credible:

Does the author, group of authors, or organization who reported this information have training and experience working in this field?	Yes	No
Is the information from a professional organization's website, book, or research article?	Yes	No
Are at least 3 on-topic references listed?	Yes	No
Was the information reported within the past 10 years?	Yes	No

The more yeses you have, the more credible the information is likely to be. The more nos you have, the less credible the source.

WHY? THEORIES ON WHY A SINGLE HAND DIFFERENCE HAPPENS

Frustratingly, there are theories, but the verifiable science at the time of this writing is suggestive but not truly known. Scientists currently are closely studying details of limb formation and regeneration of fish fins, fly and chicken wings, and salamander tails in animal research laboratories. Human embryo development is much more challenging to safely study. New discoveries are made in the field every day.

There are many theories of how a single isolated arm or hand might not completely form. The most compelling theory is based on how the heart branches into arteries like a tree: branches with a lesser amount of blood flow will not grow limbs to the same size or shape.

WHY? OTHER FACTORS THAT MAY CAUSE LIMB FORMATION DIFFERENCES

It's natural that as a parent you may still be wondering, maybe even in the back of your mind, if you did anything to cause your child's difference. Did you eat the wrong thing, was it smoking, or did you take a particular medication that could have caused it? The answer is that it's not likely. So far as we know from research, sometimes these things just happen for no reason that can be found.

Current research on factors affecting hand development can be separated into 2 groups: part 1 is *intrinsic*, the individual and combined maternal and paternal genetics. This means understanding how parent DNA contributed to your child's genetic makeup. For example, in some cases, having one child with a genetic syndrome raises the likelihood of having another, even if neither parent has the physical difference.

The second consideration is *extrinsic,* meaning whatever risk factors the carrying parent experienced or the growing embryo was exposed to during each pregnancy. Risk factors can include high-risk pregnancies, blood clotting or bleeding, placental health such as amniotic sac stability and placental location, infections, and environmental exposures.

Intrinsic Factors

The key to understanding intrinsic factors is keeping up with the best current science that tells us why limb differences happen in the first place. If your child's hand difference is due to a gene carried by many relatives in your family, it's just as likely (about 25% to 50%) that you and the same partner might have another child with the same difference.

Through genetic testing, prospective parents can know if they carry genes that may correlate with congenital differences. If you carry a gene strongly associated with known limb differences (such as a cleft hand), then you and your partner can acknowledge that your children are likely to have a similar hand difference.

Individual genes can behave differently when combined with different partner genes. So, if you had a child with one partner and are considering having a child with a different partner, the likelihood of having a child with a hand difference may change. For example, familial polysyndactyly (extra or webbed fingers) is genetically linked and passed onto offspring about 25% to 50% of the time. If you yourself have a genetically linked hand difference or carry this gene, then it is likely to be passed to your children regardless of the partner you have. If your first partner carried the gene, then you will not pass this on to your children with additional partners. However, your additional partners may carry genes for other things that will contribute to the likelihood of having children with hand differences. And your future partners may also carry genes for other conditions not related to hand differences at all. (And sometimes, new genes occur spontaneously.)

What does all this mean? There are so many variations, combinations, and unknowns that it can be difficult to determine a yes or no answer to many of these questions. If you feel you'd like to know more about your own genetics, then set aside a few hours with your partner to meet with a geneticist. The doctor will ask lots of questions and perhaps draw blood or take a cheek swab to study your DNA. The results of this testing may give you an estimate but absolutely no guarantee of the chances of having future children with genetic hand differences.

Extrinsic Factors

Extrinsic factors are those not correlated to genetic codes. These are events or exposures that occurred during the individual development of the child including toxins, infection, bleeding, or clotting. It is most likely due to *nothing* the parent did while they were pregnant—it just happened, but it still may have been an external factor that shaped how the child developed.

Experiments in animal models with acetaminophen (Tylenol®), alcohol, cigarettes, and coffee have not been linked scientifically with changes in arm formation. Exercise, vomiting, car accidents, working too much, and eating certain foods have also not been found to cause any differences. (If you can name it, pediatric researchers have tested it!) It's unlikely that any of the things you worry you might have done during pregnancy have ever been linked scientifically to lack of limb development.

Alcohol, recreational drugs, and drugs of abuse easily cross into the fetus and predominantly affect the brain. These substances have been found to alter normal development of muscles and bones in animal and human studies. Children born with these exposures are typically low in birth weight, developmentally delayed, and have formed limbs with contractures or less function. As demonstrated by the Zika virus, infection with a virus or bacteria causing developmental differences is another focus of research with no clear findings yet reported.

In the 1970s, some mothers in Europe were prescribed a drug for morning sickness called thalidomide that was linked directly to limb differences, as well as changes to the intestines, heart, and blood vessels. However, thalidomide was taken off the market long ago in the countries that were using it and was never approved for use in the United States. Pregnant parents today would not have been exposed to it.

The FDA requires that all drug labels include specific messages related to pregnancy and breastfeeding with regard to such risk. Any medication prescribed during pregnancy likely presents a low risk, has never been linked to limb differences, and was carefully prescribed to you as its benefits were needed for your overall health.

It has not been scientifically measured yet, but communities of parents of children with hand differences often compare their pregnancies and exposures to risk and can't find any similarities. Some parents exercised and had prematurity, morning sickness, twins, trauma, placental issues, and a host of other issues, and most had totally uneventful pregnancies. This all reconfirms that the hand difference was not a result of anything the parent did or did not do during their pregnancy. Doing the work to disconnect yourself emotionally from having "caused" the limb difference in your child may take time, but rest assured that there is no science or trend that supports any link at all.

As they take a complete medical history, your doctors are likely going to ask you about the details of your pregnancy. A common question is, "Did you take any medications while you were pregnant?" This sort of question can spark fear or shame. Even though you now understand the science, you may be worried by such questions that it was something you did or a decision you made during your pregnancy that caused your child's difference.

Remember, there is no scientific evidence that supports that typical medications taken during pregnancy cause limb differences. Any person asking about a medication you took or something you did during pregnancy either has not been informed by this science or is just being thorough and inquiring about your overall health. They may just be filling out your chart; they don't mean to hurt you. However, you may feel the emotion of self-blame in that moment. When this happens, identifying the emotion can be empowering and allow you to understand your response to such questions.

As you look at the whys and hows of hand differences, sometimes the medical answer is frustrating. Give me a reason. Why did this happen? How did this happen? The answer is disappointing when it is "we don't know." However, the research is fairly clear that sometimes a developmental shift happens at the embryonic stage for no reason at all or reasons we do not yet understand.

DISCUSSION QUESTIONS

After reading about formation, classifications, and statistics, what are your thoughts?

Write down your feelings about this statement: This hand difference was not a result of anything that I did or did not do.

What kind of specific hand difference does your child have? Can you categorize it?

What has surprised you about what science currently knows about the how and why of hand differences?

TWINS

Multiple births including both identical and fraternal twins occur in about 3% of all new births worldwide and may be increasing in frequency. Factors such as family history, average older maternal age (more eggs drop at once), and fertility treatments are the likely reasons. Despite these 2 or more children coming from the same parents and being exposed to the same extrinsic factors, in some cases, limb differences occur only in 1 of the twins. Some researchers have theorized that fetal stress, blood flow, or placental and amniotic sac health may be unique risk factors in twins. For example, 1 twin is getting more blood flow or space. These are only theories, and there is no science to support that at this time.

HAVING FUTURE CHILDREN

Maybe it's time to discuss having another child or grandchild. What does having one child with a limb difference mean for future siblings? Are you wondering if a hand difference can be passed down to the next generation? Should you or your children see a geneticist or DNA specialist? Let's take these questions one baby step at a time.

Some parents who may be thinking of more children are concerned about their set of intrinsic and extrinsic factors. They might even feel that they should explore options such as in vitro fertilization, egg or sperm donors, surrogacy, or adopting a child. Know that every new pregnancy will bring with it any combination of intrinsic, extrinsic, and spontaneous factors. Your likelihood of a congenital hand difference will likely be no different than with your first child. Many limb differences currently have no known genes associated with them and cannot be tested for. The overwhelming majority of people with those limb differences do not have long-standing health complications and do not have any past or future generations with those differences. If your child's difference was due to extrinsic factors, it's extremely unlikely you'd have another child with a limb difference. A new spontaneous difference can always occur, such as a subsequent child with a unique, spontaneous genetic difference.

Family planning is exciting and can reopen some of your personal feelings about you or your child. Take the time to invest in your own health and environment. Stay away from myths and negativity. Talk to doctors, such as geneticists or your child's pediatrician or hand surgeon, to learn more or reconfirm that your child's hand difference was unrelated to anything you did or did not do during your pregnancy. Discuss these emotions with your partner, primary care doctor, obstetrician, and loved ones, and check in on unexpected new feelings that might surprise you.

If you are inspired to have more children, you'll know when you are ready. Do the work to conquer the normal anxiety around your future parenthood. Enjoy the joy, fear, and celebration of this next leap in your life's journey, and share and learn from like-minded healthy new parents in your community.

DISCUSSION QUESTIONS

Are you considering having additional children?

What things are you concerned about?

What are you excited about?

CHAPTER SUMMARY

In this chapter, we learned that:

- Hand differences happen for many reasons in many different people all over the world.
- There are known scientific models of hand growth formation and classification systems. There are lots of things we just don't know.
- There are intrinsic (genetic codes) and extrinsic (not genetic) factors of congenital hand differences that relate to having more children.
- Understanding science empowers you and your child.

Chapter 4

Hand Talk: Shaping Language to Shape Your World

In this Chapter

IN THIS CHAPTER, WE WILL LEARN:

- How to guide conversations with others about your child's hand differences
- Why language matters
- Strategies for maintaining control of conversations

WHAT DO WE MEAN WHEN WE SAY "CONGENITAL HAND DIFFERENCE"?

"Congenital hand difference" is a phrase used to describe the differences in appearance and function of fingers, hands, and arms. The word "congenital" means that this difference was present at birth, whereas "acquired" means the difference occurred after birth. Medical literature spans a huge array of terms to discuss hand differences. Some terms are specific to the diagnostic terminology, such as "symbrachydactyly" or "thrombocytopenia-absent radius," and other terms are more general, such as "hand differences" or "upper limb differences." Other terminology such as "deformities," "defects," and "disfigurement" are used in medical literature today, and they very much feel outdated. A term that has emerged in recent literature is "congenital upper limb differences." However, these can feel like a lot of strange bulky words when talking with friends and family.

"Congenital hand differences" was chosen by the authors because it is only 3 words, because of its non-medical familiarity, and because of its ability to include the entire upper extremity. Children who have a difference in their arm are likely to have a difference in their hand or no hand at all. Sometimes people like to use the word "limb difference" or "upper limb difference" to distinguish it from the legs. And sometimes families make up their own name or term for the hand difference, such as "armie."

The words we use and how we use them help create tone. They reflect what we think and what we value. When we use words with negative associations, we can communicate that the hand difference is a devalued trait, such as "deformity," "deficiency," "malformation," or "missing." Terms such as "different" or "right hand" are neutral today, and then you can move into more endearing names, such as "lefty" or "armie" or "baby hand." Take the time and try out different words to find the one your family feels most comfortable using.

In addition to words, there is a component of word order. Presently both "person-first language" and "ability-first language" word order are accepted. Person-first language comes from the idea that people are people first and their descriptors are second and will often look like this in a sentence: "child with a limb difference." Ability-first language follows the traditional flow of English sentence structure with the adjectives describing the noun and will look like this: "limb-different child." Person-first and ability-first language are both used in this book interchangeably. Try out different words and word order. Reflect on the terms you use and decide if these words are the ones that accurately reflect how you want society to view your child's hand difference.

CHOOSE YOUR LANGUAGE

As you begin to understand your child's hand difference, you're going to be ready to share your child with others. These encounters can be smooth sailing, a little bumpy, or maybe a mixture of both. Parents may feel pressure from society when they take their children out and about in the world. Strangers may stare, and others may make insensitive comments. Common things people say are, "What's wrong with that kid's hand?" or "What happened?" or "Why does your baby's hand look weird?" Terms used to describe the hand difference could be "malformation," "defect," or "deformity"—none of which are words we want to use to describe our children. Know that others are subscribing to the social standards of acceptable language and have not yet been educated on the true narrative of disability. You might not have given much thought to the language you use, but as you build a deeper understanding of your child's difference, you can guide others and your child.

SOCIAL SCRIPTS

People will observe your actions, the language you use, the assistance you provide, and the body language you display as parents. All these behaviors help develop a set of social scripts for others to follow. A social script is the combination of words and actions that we use in everyday activities. There is an understood set of words and actions to create a social dialogue and exchange. This helps provide structure for social interactions and sets a series of expected behaviors, such as boarding an airplane, going to the doctor, and going to a wedding. Each of these events has a general guideline for social interactions and roles for each setting.

The challenge with hand differences is that there is no commonly understood social script for how to interact with people with hand differences. Your child may in fact be the very first person someone has met who has a hand difference. People may become confused because they do not "know what to do." They don't know if they should help or how to help. They are likely upholding the social norms that they were taught as children. They will be looking to you for guidance.

For example, at the playground, others will see you encourage your child to explore and climb, using wrists or elbows for navigating climbing structures. You'll be there to support and protect your child but still allow independence and exploration. Others will observe and learn from you and your child that children with hand differences can in fact climb on the jungle gym and this is an option for how it looks. They will learn your strategies and likely repeat them with your child and future children they meet who have hand differences.

VOCABULARY

The most important person who needs a working vocabulary is your child. Well before your baby is able to speak they will learn words for the world around them. We teach the names for body parts, family members, toys, places, and everything else. Your baby needs to know what to call their hand. Your child will choose how to talk about their hand difference with others. This is heavily influenced by how you, as parents, talk about the difference with and around your child.

Use words to craft the messaging that best helps your child. Be mindful and intentional of the initial vocabulary you use to describe your child's hand difference. Calling your child's hand or arm "missing," "deformed," "damaged," or "diseased" can be your honest initial reaction. Moving toward positive words such as "my favorite," "superpower," "cool," "small," and "loved" will impress the importance of fun or neutral terminology on those around you. Eventually your child will echo your words. Choose your words carefully, kindly, and consciously. Every parent wants their child to have the best possible chance of succeeding in the world. You can begin that process by picking a few positive descriptive words for your baby's difference. If others, even doctors, use vocabulary you don't approve of, you have the right to insist on the words you want used when describing your child's hands.

You can shape conversations and interactions with people by being intentional about the words you choose to use and how you use them. For example, you might say, "Jo, put both arms up, and help Mommy put your favorite shirt on," or "Domani, let's wash lefty first and then righty." Others will hear you use this kind of language. Feel empowered to call out situations that are having a negative impact on your child. Practice what you might say to that friend or sibling and how you teach your child to respond.

Be willing to respond with forgiveness when people say negative things without thinking. For example, a coach might say without thinking, "Alright Ash, give me a double high five." Most people struggle to know how to talk about physical differences until we help them. With education, awareness, and practice, these negative interactions will decrease. People can become more aware of and more comfortable with limb differences as they learn how to talk about them.

MAKING INTRODUCTIONS

You, as parents, get to control how and when you want to share your child's hand difference. You get to control the vocabulary you use and how you want people to interact with your child. Model these behaviors and don't be afraid to kindly redirect conversations and behavior of others as needed.

Friends and family may engage in the social script of "congratulations on having a baby, 10 fingers 10 toes" to somehow confirm that the baby is "healthy." This is not a helpful social script as it implies that all babies have 10 fingers and 10 toes, that a baby who does not fit this description has something "wrong with them," and that having something "wrong" is bad.

Your friends and family are likely not intentionally aware of these stigmas. They are merely upholding the social norms they were taught. This social script can be changed, and you can be in control of that communication. You can share something like, "Our baby is bright and beautiful and a bundle of joy." This does not imply "good" or "bad" or "healthy" or "unhealthy."

The hand difference is a part of your child and does not directly correlate to "bad."

As a parent of a child with a hand difference, you don't owe anything to anyone. If you do not want to talk about it, you have the power to end the discussion, especially in daily interactions. A lengthy conversation about your new baby will not deepen the relationship you have with the person behind you in line at the post office. You are not responsible for other people's feelings. Be who you are and enjoy the things you want to do. Let others adapt on their own, even if those having a hard time processing the difference are your friends and family.

If the person making the inappropriate comments is a child, you can correct and educate them. But if it continues, you can control your space. You can say things like, "We use the term 'armie' to describe our child's hand, and we would appreciate it if you used these terms too," or "Let's try that again. 'Deformed' has a negative connotation and is not necessarily a word we want to use to describe ourselves. What are other words we can use that can be more kind?" or simply "Let's try that again." It may feel uncomfortable to engage in this type of education. Feel free to practice saying these responses or role play with friends and family. The more you practice it, the more naturally it will come in conversations.

DISCUSSION QUESTIONS

What was your first experience bringing your new baby to an event with new people?

What was it like to introduce your child?

What is something that you were proud of in your introduction?

What is something, if anything, you wish were better?

How do you want the next interaction to go?

FAMILY AND FRIENDS

Know that you also can talk with family members about the language you and your child want used. You can talk with them about how you are teaching your child to interact with objects. You might have to explain to your relatives that you like to use humor, for example, joking that the hand was "bitten off by a shark" when describing your child's hand to new people. You can work to include family members and request that they respect you and your child by using the language and strategies you use with immediate family. Extended family can be an influential and positive support system around a child with hand differences.

It's most important to remember that this is the beginning of the conversation, a chance to open and try on different ways of communicating with your family and world. This may feel different as your family grows older, and maybe you will revisit it over the years with different lenses and perspectives. Feel empowered to explore topics further. Social interactions are complex and layered and can be exhausting. Forgive yourselves and learn from less than ideal reactions or conversations with friends and family. This is an ever-evolving process.

DISCUSSION QUESTIONS

Reflect on when you first shared your child to everyone you know and love through a birth announcement.

How did you feel?

What was that process like?

How did others respond?

USING SOCIAL SCRIPTS

You have the freedom to develop the social scripts that work best for your family. You may find some are better for your child when meeting other kids for the first time. Or you may find your child likes them for interacting with unfamiliar people who seem to stare or make comments. As they grow, your child can decide what words they want to use to describe themselves, what stories they want to tell, and how much of their story they want to tell. Children are not required to explain themselves if they do not want to—and it's important to let them know that. We repeat, children do not need to explain their hand difference if they do not want to. They get to decide who they trust and if they want to accept them into their own circle of friends.

DISCUSSION QUESTIONS

Reflect on social interactions and meeting new or unfamiliar people.

What has the conversation about your child's hand difference been so far?

Have they asked questions?

How have you responded?

How has your child responded?

Do you have a "go-to" explanation, and what is included in it?

What do you like about the interactions you are having so far?

What do you wish you could change?

Responses can include humor or expanded education, or be simple and sweet. You can use techniques like writing, drawing, or story development to help your family express how they want to communicate. This group effort can be helpful for siblings and extended family as well. Going through this process helps your child understand that they are in control of their story and how they want to share it.

Let's look at some simple scripts. As you learn some examples to get you started, you'll see many more you'd like to add. You can begin with these basic scripts and adapt them or build your own. The key is to use vocabulary as a tool to help send the messages you and your child want received.

Introducing Themselves

CHILD: *"Hi, my name is Zary. This is what my hand looks like. I can do the things that I need to do and want to do, it just might look different, and that's OK! I really like to play basketball. Want to see how I shoot a basket? Lemme show you!"*

Responding to Questions

QUESTIONS: "*What happened?*" or "*Why does your (arm/hand/finger) look like that?*"

CHILD:

1. Short: "*I was born this way.*"
2. Humor: "*It was bitten off by a shark.*"
3. Little detail: "*When I was born, I didn't have fingers, and at 5 years old I had a surgery that made me a thumb.*"

At any point children can say:

"*That's really all I have to say, thanks for asking.*"

"*I don't have anything to say right now.*"

"*I don't want to talk about it right now. Thank you for understanding.*"

Your child can choose the language they want to when talking about their limb difference and can help request that others use this language:

"*I like to use the word 'limb difference,' and it shows me respect when you use this word too.*"

"*I call this my 'armie.' You can call it armie, too.*"

Your child can choose to answer or not answer questions that may be asked of them or can explore ways of sharing their experiences with others. Further examples include:

"*I don't do that the way you do, but let me show you how I can.*"

From a parent: "*He doesn't do that the way you do, but he is very good at figuring things out.*"

If the child does not know the answer they can say:

"*I don't have the answer to that. Let's go to the playground.*"

"*I don't know, but let's go ask the teacher (my dad, your mom, etc.).*"

And end with, "*Let's go play.*"

If the child has had surgery, they can show a scar and state:

"*I had an operation, but I don't remember because I was too little. Have you ever had an operation?*"

Feel free to role play with your child, especially when entering a transition (new school, new grade, new sports team, summer camps, new club) or anytime there is a wide group of new people and best friends, siblings, or cousins may not be attending the same events. These social scripts are helpful to address and understand new prosthetic devices, medical equipment, casts/splints, or medical interventions.

Your child may feel better prepared to enter new situations when practicing explanations. Depending on how your family communicates, you all may choose to write a song or make a picture or create a story. Your child can use this story, song, or drawing to facilitate communication in a new setting.

DISCUSSION QUESTIONS

Let's build a practice social script.

1. Write down a hypothetical situation, such as attending the first day at school, practicing for the first time with a new sports team, or meeting another family on the playground.
2. Write down a comment you might receive from one of the individuals in your hypothetical situation.
3. Describe different responses that could address this comment, such as ones that use humor, are short, or go into detail.

Use this format to plan out conversations with different situations.

NAVIGATING QUESTIONS

There are a number of children's books about limb-different characters. Some are written by limb-different authors and their families. You can find them by searching for "limb difference" when talking with your librarian or bookstore associate, or on a renting/shopping website. Having them available for children and family members to read can be useful. Via these books, you can help support strong and positive communications about limb differences. Your child may not want to or may not know how to have a direct conversation with you, but they might pick up a book or let you read it to them as a bedtime story. As they see themselves in the characters, they can feel empowered to take better control of how they communicate about their limb difference.

BULLYING

At some point, your child is likely to have a negative interaction. As much as we wish that we live in a fully understanding society, people will make comments that may not be meant to be hurtful, but are. Or, sadly, people may make comments that are in fact intended to be hurtful. It's important to practice navigating these situations as a family, too. How can you best address and respond to these comments?

When interacting with negative descriptions from others about the upper limb difference, try these phrases in response:

QUESTION: *"So you were born deformed?"*
RESPONSE: *"Let's try that again. I like to say 'hand difference,' not 'deformed,' when talking about my hand. It shows me respect when you say 'hand difference' too."*

When it comes to negative experiences, children may share the experiences with adults they trust. Parents and adults listening to their story can ask reflective questions to help change this type of interaction in the future. Try to focus on questions that help explore feelings like, "How did that make you feel?" or "What did you want to happen?" and "How can we make this a better situation in the future?" These kinds of questions can spark discussions helping the child feel valued and respected. They also help them to feel more in control of the interactions and less helpless in the conversation. If your child responds well but shares that they experience anxiety in the moment, then you can move beyond the script into understanding their feelings to help them regain control of the situation. Your child can establish boundaries about what they want to share and can ask for others to respect their choices.

Trusted adults can also role play with children, allowing them to develop and practice words and situations as needed. We encourage forms of expression via writing, drawing, performance, or anything that is a creative outlet for children to express their experiences.

Be mindful of your child's behaviors and ask probing questions if you suspect or if you become aware of a bullying interaction at a space where the bully and your child frequent often, such as school or extra-curricular classes. If you suspect events are happening, you can ask your child, "Who is your best friend at school today?" or "Who did you play with at recess?" If the child has a hard time answering these questions, shift to, "Who is a mean (bad or naughty) kid at school?" and "What makes them mean?" If you notice that your child has a hard time sharing positive interactions but very easily shares negative interactions, you as a parent have the legal right to discuss with school administration. Your child has the legal right to school and meaningful activities. If bullying is impacting their success and enjoyment in these spaces, it may be necessary to intervene. Legal protections are discussed further in Chapter 11.

DISCUSSION QUESTIONS

What have you noticed when your child meets new children?

What did you say?

What did your child say or do?

What did the other kids say or do?

What things have surprised you?

What strategies worked well for you and for your child?

What things can be improved, if anything?

When it comes to navigating friends, social situations, and societal expectations, it's important to provide a safe space for your child to express themselves as needed. Let them be the leaders in the conversation and be respectful of their wants and wishes. Allow them to explore the activities that give them meaning instead of superimposing what you think they should say or do because of your own fears or insecurities. Really be mindful of yourself and your coping mechanisms.

SOCIAL SCRIPTS FOR SCHOOL

As your child enters school, you may want to talk through a variety of new situations with them, especially if they have some concerns about meeting new people. Spontaneously searching for words can be difficult at times, and children may find it beneficial to have a series of social scripts for the school setting. Now that your child is entering school, they may want to build on these preestablished scripts or pull out and practice the scripts that are most applicable for the school setting. Social scripts can be helpful as you encounter various new situations with your child and help them find words they want to use. Introductions and interacting with new children may be the most difficult or the easiest when your child is young, as they are still learning how to navigate things.

As children age, they may begin to have these types of conversations with teachers, coaches, youth group leaders, and summer camp counselors on their own. While they gain confidence, work to develop a relationship where they feel confident asking for assistance in building and navigating these conversations. Over time, you may find that your child has a particular person they like to ask for guidance in communicating. It might be you or your partner, a trusted friend, a family member, a counselor, or other health care professionals.

CHAPTER SUMMARY

In this chapter, we learned:

- How to determine the language your family wants to use
- How to develop social scripts
- How to develop strategies for navigating conversations about your child's hand difference
- How to develop ways for your child to end conversations
- That you are not responsible for anyone's feelings and can end conversations at any time

Part II
Health Care

Chapter 5

Getting the Most out of Doctor Appointments and Opinions

In this Chapter

IN THIS CHAPTER, WE WILL LEARN:

- To prepare to learn about the medical, therapeutic, and prosthetic options for your child
- To stay organized as you learn
- To appreciate that some medical care options are time dependent, and decisions may need to be made on behalf of your child, to the best of your ability

GETTING ORGANIZED

As the parent of a child with a congenital hand difference, you may want to keep track of medical records, second opinions, internet information, and school paperwork at times. We recommend that you take a minute to create an organization system. This helps you feel empowered and prepared to manage medical decisions. Everything can be important in the beginning, including where you keep the writings of your own thoughts and feelings.

This organization can be a physical system like a binder or an accordion-style portable filing folder with hard copies of insurance forms and your notes. More portably, it can be an electronic system like an organizational file app or a folder on your desktop, in a shared drive, or in the cloud. Regardless of which you choose, it's important you create a system that works for you to quickly access needed forms and medical records.

For making a physical system, a simple trip to the office supply store (or a few clicks at your favorite online shopping site) will help you find the info you need to get organized. If you choose an electronic system, a smartphone, laptop, or tablet may be all you need. Here are some additional tips for success:

- **Organize in a way that makes sense to you.** Create a careful organization system, such as page dividers for easy access to each document at a moment's notice. Subsections could include general medical records, surgical notes, therapy reports, prosthetic prescriptions and vendors, school assessments, copies of x-rays, lists of medications and allergies, and family contact information for emergencies. Bookmark, print, or save copies of information you may want to reference or read again.
- **Bring your files with you.** We recommend bringing with you to all appointments either the physical files or a device with access to the electronic ones. Use this to add new information your health care providers share with you and your child. Ask your health care team for a copy of the notes they wrote during the session, and store this copy in your organizational system. Ask health care providers to spell words that you want to look up later for your own research and add in this new information. Create a list of questions you want to ask your providers, and bring this sheet to your meeting to ensure that all your questions are answered.
- **Mark your notes before you go.** Don't be afraid to create starred, flagged, or highlighted sections or use sticky notes on sections that are most relevant in each document. Highlight passages you'd like to research more fully or ask your partner or a family member to read.
- **Don't forget to bring a pen/notetaking device to the appointment.** Make sure you always have a backup pen or pencil for an appointment or the ability to add to the electronic file notes. If you are 2 adults, designate 1 of you to take notes in advance. You can then add notes from each visit like a journal: what happened, what the care team ordered, what they said, and what action steps you and your child may need to take before the next appointment. Make a habit of taking your system with you to appointments as needed and updating it with new documents and notes when you visit doctors and other medical professionals. Sometimes, it can be hard to absorb information when your mind is busy with what this all means. Having it written down makes it easy to refer to later on and can make it easy to cross reference with other health care professionals.

You can add worksheets and journal pages for your thoughts or discussion questions from this book. Add a calendar and set milestones and check-ins for yourself. You can include the status checks from Chapter 1 to see how you're doing compared to the month prior. As you answer each question, look back at past worksheets, notes, or lists you've made, and see what has changed. Before you know it, the organization will have you feeling more empowered and more in control of experiences like obtaining new medical information or meeting a new doctor, therapist, or prosthetist. As your child grows up, you can pass along this organizational system when they start taking the lead on their medical appointments.

- **Add medical records, x-rays, and advanced imaging along the way.** Some of your medical records may need to be requested through the medical records office. When you request a file, they will print it for you, send you an electronic file, or burn you a CD. Make sure you can open it and add it to your organized system. It is best to keep these updated along the way. If you move locations or seek second opinions and years go by, it can take hours of phone calls to get through to someone to send them to you.

BUILDING YOUR CHILD'S HEALTH CARE TEAM

There are many roles within health care, and many potential members of the team you may work with. Let's introduce some professionals you may interact with and review their roles.

Pediatrician or Family Practitioner

A pediatrician is typically the main doctor overseeing your child's general health. Having this doctor know more about your child than anyone else gives a strong point of contact for future needs and referrals. They will be aware of hand differences but likely do not have specialty in this area. This doctor will be your home base. They will make referrals, recommend testing, and interpret results. They'll also conduct your well-child exams over time. Creating a strong and trusting relationship with this doctor is recommended, as the child's needs may change with time.

Medical Specialists

Geneticist: If your child's hand difference is genetic or hereditary, you might see a geneticist. A geneticist is a doctor who specializes in genetic testing of DNA and interpreting results. You might also work with a genetics nurse, a nurse specially trained in working with patients on treatment plans based on the results of genetic testing. A geneticist will be able to tell you if your child's hand difference is genetically linked and the likelihood that future siblings will also have hand differences.

Other specialists: If your child's hand difference is not their only difference, they may need to see other specialists. Cardiologists (heart), nephrologists (kidney), and hematologists (blood cells) are just a few of the specialists sometimes but not always involved in the care of children with hand differences. Typically, the pediatrician will need to make a referral, and some of these specialists will be in or out of your network. Waiting for appointments for specialists can take time and will be made urgent by your pediatrician only if needed.

Hand Surgeons

Hand surgeons care for patients with congenital and acquired hand differences as well as arthritis and traumatic injuries to hands. You should make sure your surgeon is board certified by the orthopedic, plastic surgery, or general surgery board. This information is typically on the website of the certifying board in each field but can be researched by the surgeon's state medical licensing as well. An additional Subspecialty Certificate in Surgery of the Hand is awarded only to those surgeons who have done further specialty training at US-accredited programs in caring specifically for human hands. Your surgeon should have had extra training or focus on the child's hand (versus the adult hand).

Hand surgery may be completed by different kinds of surgeons. There can be some overlap and some more specific skill sets in doctors of orthopedic surgery, general surgery, and plastic surgery. Any of these surgical specialties can be a path to specialized congenital hand surgery training. Each surgeon may be qualified to be your child's doctor for different reasons.

As you are reviewing options with the doctors on your care team, make sure you understand why your child was referred to a particular kind of surgeon. Ask each specialist what qualifies them to guide treatment decisions in your child's care, and this will likely lead you to the correct one. As limb differences are rare, some surgeons will have more experience than others. Simply talking with them will give you the best answers.

Prosthetists

Prosthetists are health care providers that work with your child to evaluate, fabricate, and fit assistive devices for the activities your child wants to do.

There are a wide variety of prosthetic devices, and developing a strong relationship with the prosthetist will allow you to ask a lot of questions, ensure the device is fitting properly, ensure the device is working effectively for your child, or confirm if you need to come in for repairs. Most urban areas or regional care centers are home to groups of technicians who specialize in upper limb prosthetics. It is likely worth visiting one of these to find up-to-date technology and options. Prosthetics are a referred specialty, and you will need a prescription from a physician (your pediatrician or your hand surgeon) to meet with a prosthetist. This is worth a conversation with your insurance company and your prosthetist to determine what options are available and what devices might work best for your family.

Therapists

There are several types of therapists who may work with your child. Typically, therapists will schedule multiple sessions over a set time period and will work toward specific goals developed with your child.

Physical therapists (PTs) and occupational therapists (OTs) are a part of the rehabilitation team. PTs have an approach to increase strength and range of motion, which is accomplished through exercise and movement. OTs have an approach to increase access to the activities people need and want to do throughout their days. This is managed through increasing strength, increasing range of motion, finding adaptive skills, using adaptive equipment, and modifying environments for people to do activities.

Counseling therapists, psychologists, and social workers can work with your child to develop supports and strategies for supporting mental health. Your child may have therapists in a school setting who will provide support related to engagement in school-based activities, whereas they may have other therapists in a hospital or rehabilitation setting who target activities more related to self-care.

Nurses and Physician Assistants

Nurses and physician assistants are likely to work alongside the doctor to ensure that all your needs are met when interacting with the health care system. Nurses and/or physician assistants may be easier to communicate to or spend a more significant amount of time with your family and your child providing pre- and postoperative care. They can even provide support to the family if you're in the hospital for a longer stay. They can also be a prominent part of your care team with in-home care.

Healers and Care Team Members

You may have additional people you consider part of your care team. Chiropractors, acupuncturists, massage therapists, or even nontraditional healers may be on your child's care team. These fields are less well-regulated than other types of medicine, and some practitioners may have extensive knowledge of hand differences while others won't. However, as with any member of your circle of care, they may be effective for your child, you, and your family.

As with all health care providers, seek out those with experience with children similar to your child. These costs typically are not covered by insurance and may be considered out-of-pocket. Ask for references. Consider reputation and reviews. Be mindful of in-network and out-of-network practitioners.

NAVIGATING HEALTH CARE TEAMS

Think back on the day you discovered the hand news and the initial diagnosis of your child's hand difference. Who was the health care professional that diagnosed the hand difference? What is their background? Do they specialize in kids' hands? Have you considered a second opinion just to ensure you have explored any options? Don't be afraid to challenge a diagnosis if you want clarity and confirmation that this is the correct diagnosis. Accurate diagnosis is important for caring for your child's overall health, and there is a discrete usefulness to having the correct name to describe the hand difference.

As you meet new team members, pay attention to their engagement. If they are not supportive or helpful, you may need to find someone new. It's OK to limit contact from people who create negative feelings for you. If members of your care team generate anxiety or blame instead of positive, healthy relationships, consider changing them.

When working with your care team, there are a few approaches you can use to be successful. For example:

- Have a good handle on how to discuss your pregnancy and birth events.
- Make a list of questions to ask at each appointment and write the answers down. When you are nervous or stressed, you might not remember what the doctor said clearly, so having notes can be useful.
- Make sure you communicate if there were any medical conditions that affected your pregnancy or events during pregnancy or birth that will become part of you and your child's health profile.
- Write down the language and terms you want your health care team to use and ask them to use the preferred language.

DISCUSSION QUESTIONS

Reflect on interactions with your care team.

Who made you feel stressed?

Which individuals made you feel safe? Did you feel empowered to say something to this person?

Did you change caregivers?

What action did you take (or can you take) to make yourself feel more supported and heard?

There will be times that you are frustrated, anxious, or grateful, so feel empowered to communicate that. Feel free to ask questions, confirm details, write down their recommendations, and remember that together, you are all on a team for your child.

THINKING AHEAD ABOUT MEDICAL DECISIONS

When it comes to medical interventions or treatments, options can get confusing, so it might help to think of a menu with sections like surgery, prosthetics, and therapies. The interventions menu provides you and your child with options for using their hand difference from day to day. For example, within the same day, a child may tie shoes with one hand in the morning, play baseball with a sports prosthetic arm in the afternoon, and decide to go to a social event wearing a bionic arm in the evening. Another child may choose to gain the ability to use their hand in a way they could not prior to surgery. Yet another may decide to have more surgeries ahead, and current functionality isn't what it eventually will be.

As you learn about the options to help your child navigate daily life, you are probably exploring a number of paths including therapy, surgical options, and prosthetics. This sort of fluidity creates a constant exploration of what an individual with a hand difference wants and needs when it comes to typical goals of independence, capability, and even appearance. These options will change over the course of your child's growth.

When children are younger, parents may be taking on a majority of the decision making for their child. Some medical decisions will naturally and thoughtfully be made before the child can meaningfully participate. As children get older, engaging them with decision making becomes possible. Let them make their own choices as they're old enough to understand what they might like. Research shows that kids around 8 to 9 years old can make solid choices on their preferred medical treatments when they are given information about treatment options that is developmentally appropriate to them. As your child grows and develops unique preferences, these wants and needs may change, too. Although treatment options can seem overwhelming, research suggests that the quality of a child's life is unlikely to be set by any one of these interventions any more than their natural skills and talents, grit, dreams, environment, community, friends and family, and experience of emotional coping.

Some of the sections of the menu are time dependent, such as operations that take advantage of future growth potential, and won't be available or as easily integrated into function later. Feeling as if you're choosing for your child can make decisions even more challenging. You may have to decide for your child without knowing what they would have wanted for themselves.

We acknowledge that this is a tough choice. Surgeries at a young age will determine how a child learns to grasp and pinch. It's a little bit like learning a new language. Younger children pick up new languages much more quickly if you introduce them at a very young age. They simply learn it more easily than if a language is introduced later. Once they have defined ways of communicating or functioning, it's harder for them to learn new ones.

DISCUSSION QUESTIONS

Has surgery been presented to your family? If so, what are the surgical options?

What goals do you have for your child?

What goals does your child have for themselves?

What goals does your partner or co-parent have for your child?

What goals does your surgeon have?

Are these goals all the same or are they different?

Which surgery you choose (or refuse) does not determine your child's future, but it may determine function. To use the language analogy, a surgery determines the language they will speak, not the ability to speak at all. Does it feel like you are deciding something that could change their life? As a parent, these feelings are natural. There is no right answer, but you can choose what's best for your child based on the information you have today.

Regardless of which menu options you choose, it's important to gather as much research as you need to feel empowered in your choice. By learning as much as you can, you can make an educated decision knowing that the right choice for your child may be different than for other kids. Understand that it is also impossible to know everything. Parents have made lots of medical decisions that they and their children are satisfied with years later without knowing all of the details.

To help you get started, we've outlined some basic menu categories in the next few chapters with ideas of what you might find in each section. Be aware that when you talk to other parents and people with hand differences, they have made their own choices for their own reasons. Listen to their stories, ask lots of questions, and remember that a lot of people have very strong and conflicting emotions on these topics. Every child and every family is unique, and you know what is best for your family and for your child. No one else can or should make these decisions for you.

Know that sometimes menu options are unavailable, not recommended, or not physically possible depending on the formation of the hand difference. For example, thumb-making is not possible unless wrist bones are present, so it isn't an option if the forearm is absent below the elbow. Be sure to talk with your surgeon, who can tell you what is feasible and safe for your child specifically. Doctors will know older children and adults who have had similar types of surgeries when they were younger and will know about how they function as they grow. Surgeons will base recommendations for your family on their skill set, understanding, research, and experience. Therefore, different surgeons may offer different options. Feel empowered to meet with a variety of surgeons to see what options are recommended from each surgeon. This is a good thing.

DISCUSSION QUESTIONS

Talking with others about your choices for your child can be difficult. As you talk with others, you'll quickly find there are words or phrases that seem unsupportive of your decision, such as "you must" or "you should not."

What are some phrases you don't want to hear?

Describe a situation where someone's unwelcoming speech made you feel unsupported.

What changes have you made in your own language when talking about treatment decisions?

CHAPTER SUMMARY

In this chapter, we learned:

- That there can be many members of the health care team, and each plays a role in supporting your family and your child
- That there are several options for choosing treatments and interventions for your child
- To make medical decisions that feel right for you and your child based on current goals for your child. Those goals will change over time.
- That communication and being empowered to choose the members of your care team are strategies that most likely will result in positive relationships

Chapter 6

Hand Surgery: Indications and Techniques

In this Chapter

IN THIS CHAPTER, WE WILL LEARN:

- Surgical options for changing the form and function of hands with differences
- Surgical techniques, how they work, and what may determine the potential procedure for your child
- Expected outcomes, benefits, and risks of surgery

Perhaps this is the very first chapter you decide to read or the very last. Parents of children with hand differences express general curiosity as well as initially firm beliefs as to whether surgery is the first option they want to know about. There are many surgical options available, some of which may be an option for your child. Medical science can't yet grow your child a new hand. But depending on your child's age and hand difference, there may be ways to change the appearance of the hand or increase your child's hand use and functionality.

Surgery on the hands of children is conducted every day worldwide, and surgeons have trained in these fields for years with plenty of protocols and policies created to protect your child. Anesthesia technology has advanced to ensure your child is comfortable and safe while having their surgery. No surgery will be a guarantee and all will have some risk. If the goal is to change the form or function of the child's limb, you may consider these surgical risks.

Modern medicine universities and corporations are conducting research studies on stem cells and umbilical cord blood and how one person's body can accept the tissue of another person without serious risk. And while science can do some pretty cool things, it still isn't able to give a child a replacement hand or arm like Luke Skywalker's amazingly real forearm full of bionic parts. It is still unlikely that a surgical intervention will create a typical-looking hand. Science will continue to make advances yet already today can offer your child a wide variety of useful options for changing the form and function of hand differences in children.

In this chapter we will discuss surgery of a child's hand in extensive detail. Skin incisions and flaps will describe how the skin can be moved around to change the way the hand looks or works. We will review the role of temporary and permanent hardware, such as internal and external devices (metal plates, screws, wires, pins, and fixators). We will discuss how skin and bones can be straightened, lengthened, or even transferred from one area of the body to another. There is a lot of information in this section. Take it in as slowly or as quickly as you like, depending on your comfort with surgical descriptions.

Many people want to think of surgery as a cure-all. It's in our nature as well as most cultural systems to believe that medicine or surgeons can "fix" and heal. After all, surgeons work miracles every day, right? When it comes to the severity and nature of your child's difference, a surgeon may indeed be able to improve the form and function or may not have any options to offer at all. The ultimate measure of a successful surgery will be if it increases your child's ability to function in a confident and independent way.

Surgery to your child's hand can change the *how* of what your child will accomplish. It won't change the *if* of what they are able to accomplish when it comes to being happy and healthy. People born with no fingers at all can type on a keyboard and play the piano and become doctors, musicians, athletes, models, and mechanics and can achieve enormous successes in their chosen fields. These children will grow as humans experiencing all the emotional and physical aspects of life. What surgery they had when they were young will have something, *but not everything*, to do with how they cope, adapt, and thrive.

Surgical terms can be overwhelming. They're long and hard to say or spell, and many words can be used to describe the same thing. You may have an emotional or physical reaction to the terms or description of the surgery. Take the time to learn the procedure name your surgeon is recommending. Write it down. Learn to spell it. When you face something straight on it becomes less frightening in the long run. You can look it up and research it. Learn the expected outcome, and understand it and the risks you are taking as well as the benefits it could have for your child. See if you can be connected to others who have it and learn what their experiences have been.

FORM AND FUNCTION SURGICAL INTERVENTIONS

Specific surgeries focus on creating form and function out of the limb that's already there, such as separating webbed fingers, straightening or lengthening arms or fingers, or adding or rotating small amounts of bone or skin. Other procedures focus on creating function by significantly altering the hand from what it was, such as moving whole toes to the hand. We will review some general categories of surgeries and surgical techniques. Form and function surgeries may involve many combined procedures at once, such as adding skin after separating fingers.

INCISIONS, SKIN FLAPS, GRAFTS, AND SCARS

Surgeries leave scars and skin color differences, especially if skin was moved from one part of the body to another. It is important to work with your surgeon and your child to understand what those scars will look like. Each person will scar and heal differently, and oftentimes scarring can be difficult to predict.

Skin is an organ, and if you keep its life force with it, you can rotate it, pick it up, move it around, and reattach it someplace else. The simplest of ways to manipulate skin involves skin flaps. Skin flaps are created by making zigzag incisions leaving the skin in triangles but still attached on 1 side. Moving the skin around in triangles is a wonderful geometry not too dissimilar from working with cloth. These skin flaps are commonly used in syndactyly surgeries and z-plasties.

Why is there a *Z* in the procedure "z-plasty"? If you take the letter *Z* and create 2 triangles in the skin that make up the letter and keep them attached, the triangles can be rearranged into the shape of a letter *N*. This will increase the width of a space in the "web" between the fingers or release a tight contracture—which is stiff or shortened skin—while still leaving everything covered. It is a wonderful tool to reconstruct the hand when needed. When a few *Z*'s are lined up next to each other, it's called multiple z-plasties.

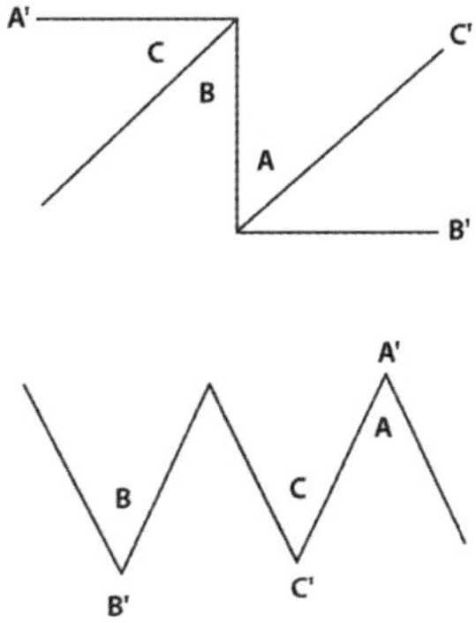

Figure 6-1: Skin flaps in a z-plasty that redistribute skin in triangles to increase length at the expense of width.

When the skin can't be rearranged or rotated, it can be brought from a totally different part of the body. Since the life force (blood vessels, nerves, etc.) is separated, these transfers are more complex. If the receiving area is well-prepared, the body will accept it and slowly assimilate it because it wants to be covered by skin. There are several types of skin grafts.

Full-Thickness Skin Grafts

A full-thickness skin graft is one where all the layers of skin are taken from an area big enough that extra skin won't be missed. You can take a graft from anywhere you can pinch skin and the area would still be covered without the skin inside the pinch. Although skin could be taken from anywhere, much thought is put into where the best skin for the hand might come from and where the scar will be least noticeable. This procedure is used for syndactyly surgeries and to cover areas that need skin after other surgeries. Surgeons work to match skin as best as possible. For example, if the surgeon performs a circumcision at the same time as the hand surgery, the foreskin can serve as a full-thickness skin graft. However, the nature, elasticity, and coloring of the harvested skin will remain. If the skin is harvested from someplace that is pink or dark or grows hair, that may happen in the new location.

One good place for small skin donor sites can be from the crease on the inside of the wrist, as it heals in a straight line and the scar can look like a natural crease. Other potential donor sites are from the outside edge of the hand or the soft front of the elbow. When lots of skin is needed, some surgeons use the groin or lower belly. Sometimes skin transplanted from these areas may darken with time or even grow hair. Depending on how much is needed, that might be the most convenient location. Skin lighteners or hair removal can be pursued later if the appearance would benefit.

Split-Thickness Skin Graft

Another option is a split-thickness graft where surgeons take large areas of the top layer of skin cells, typically from the front of the thigh. They leave enough layers so that the donor area can regrow, although it will leave a scar. (It might look like a scrape that's healed.) The transplanted layer can then be placed over an area that needs skin. The skin will assimilate, although it will always have a texture or look like it has been scarred. This technique is used a lot for burn surgeries where large areas of the body need to be covered in new skin.

Patches of skin for transfers may come from organ donors, come from animals, or be grown in a lab. In the future, skin cells might even come in a spray. Fortunately, the skin grafts needed for hand surgeries are typically small. Surgeons will use these options to cover any area in need. Anywhere there is skin surgery, there will be scarring, and that may affect the finger as it grows.

Syndactyly or Webbing Release Surgery

When a child's hand forms differently, fingers can be small or webbed, attached to each other, or even stacked on top of each other, all united with skin. Any combination of this difference when it comes to fingers is called partial or complete finger syndactyly.

If each finger has its own bones, nerve, and arteries, the connected fingers can be fully separated by a surgeon. Because fingers bend and even move a little bit side to side, the surgery needs to be done carefully to give the new skin around the fingers the flexibility it needs. Surgeons rearrange the available skin and use various methods to patch bare spots, creating unique zigzag scars that are not straight lines. This is the z-plasty. The zigzag scars heal thinner and allow for more finger motion than straight line scars. Scars will fade as the child ages; however, they will likely remain visible.

With syndactyly release, each finger needs its own skin, so when separating the digits, the surgeon may need additional skin to cover each finger. The surgeon becomes sort of a tailor with the skin, like making pants out of a skirt. If you put 2 fingers together and then separate them, you can see all the new skin that would be needed to cover the inner surface of each separated finger. Skin to cover these new openings may need to come from another part of the body, as described above, with a full thickness skin graft.

Fingernails that are joined can be separated, too, although this operation can be challenging to get just right. Often, the nails that need separating are not straight or round to begin with and may be thicker or thinner than other nails. If the first surgery doesn't get the nail quite right, it can be tolerated, the nail can be removed, or additional surgeries can be attempted later should you or your child find them beneficial.

These surgeries are all currently done with stitching, needle, and surgical thread called "suture," just like a tailor, to attach the new skin and connect the edges together. Surgeons use specific kinds of stitches or thread materials for stitching that the body will absorb and won't need removal. After surgery, the surgeon will put the child in a cast or splint to keep the area safe, clean, and dry. Sometimes a care team professional will change the dressing a few times. For children, most surgeons use rapidly self-dissolving or absorbable suture material rather than ones

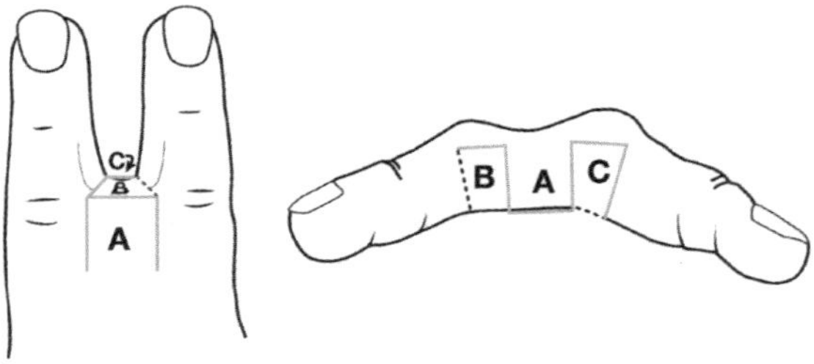

Figure 6-2: Webbed fingers (syndactyly). During surgery, skin can be moved around in flaps to create webspaces that are soft and natural. Areas from which that skin was removed may need to be covered by skin grafts.

you'd have to take out after a few weeks. Absorbable stitches heal into a scab which will gradually fall off when the fingers are unwrapped and washed.

Underneath these scabs there will be new, pink, healthy skin. The new area will need special scar care and protection from sun exposure until it is soft and pliable. As a parent, you can massage the scar to help keep it soft. Softer scars will stretch with the child as they grow and give a better cosmetic result. Scar massage is a deep tissue massage with ultra-hydrating creams that will help prevent scar tissue from becoming stuck to the tendons or joints under the skin layer, thickening, or turning darker. It can be taught to you and later to the child to improve scar appearance. More on scars in the skin grafts and flaps section.

If the child has syndactyly surgery or web releases while they are young, your doctor will want to monitor the growth of the fingers over time. With growth, the hand can change, and scars can thicken in between the fingers. They can also become a little less straight or create nail irregularities. These can be addressed with additional surgeries should your child want them or if these differences are negatively impacting function. If the fingers did not bend prior to the surgery because they didn't have joints or tendons, then they most likely won't bend after the surgery either, but will move side to side better once separated.

Digit or Arm Lengthening Surgery

Sometimes the fingers (also called digits), forearm, or upper arm are incompletely formed or are shorter or thinner than expected. It is possible to lengthen these bones. It is also possible to move small bones from the toes (leaving the toe itself a little wigglier) into the hand and sometimes, but not always, lengthening them. This surgery is used most when there is a nubbin without bone or a partial finger that could be lengthened to help the child pinch or grip. It can also be performed when the forearm is too short for a prosthesis with an elbow hinge component. If lengthening the forearm would help the prosthesis work better or help the child reach their world, then this surgery might be an option.

A surgeon has a few options for lengthening bones depending on the existing structure. One option is a set of pins and a bar placed in the bone and out through the skin that slowly makes the bone longer over many months. The parents turn the bar just a millimeter every day so that it doesn't hurt to stretch the arm or fingers. This gradually lengthens the bone and allows new skin to grow where needed. However, this procedure doesn't create joints, so these bones cannot bend. Lengthening a finger, for example, would create a long single bone that cannot bend (no knuckles). This can still provide function for things like grip and dexterity more effectively than the nubbins or shorter fingers a child might have been born with. Longer fingers aren't always better because they don't bend. Shorter fingers may make pinch easier, so the decision to have lengthening surgeries needs to incorporate that.

Another option is to use bone from somewhere else in the child's own body and insert it or attach it to the short bones of the hand to make it longer. Bone from the pelvis hip bone (iliac crest), knee, or toes is most common. This sort of bone

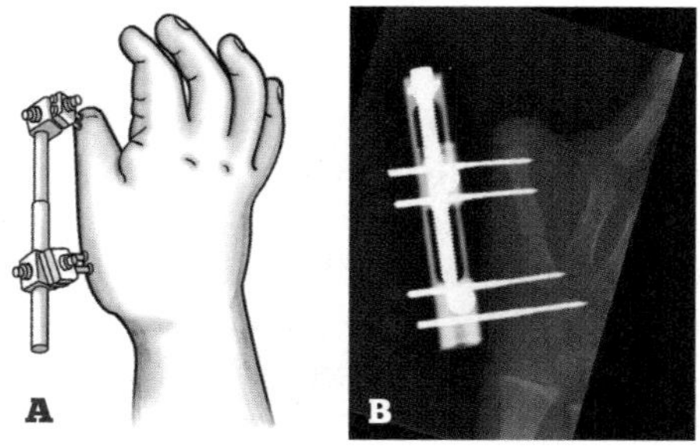

Figure 6-3 A and B: An external fixator or pin-and-bar apparatus for slowly lengthening bones over months. From the outside (A) parents will turn the bars several times a day and keep the metal clean. From the inside (B) the bone edges separate with each turn. The body can fill in this gap if the process is done approximately 1 mm per day, resulting in a solid longer bone.

moving is done all in 1 day. Therefore, skin to cover the immediate longer length of the digit must already be present. If there is not enough skin, then the slower method of gradually lengthening is suggested.

Partial Toe Bone Transfers

Without taking the whole toe, surgeons can take parts (usually bones or nails) from the toes and move them up to the hand. When a child's hand has nubbins or partially formed fingers, it is called symbrachydactyly. A hand formed in this way may even have only wiggly pieces of skin instead of fully formed digits. Surgeons can fill these types of digits with firm bones that (hopefully!) will grow as the child grows, moving just 1 bone (or phalanx) of the toe but leaving the rest of the toe in place. The strengthened, less wiggly nubbin can help the child with pinch strength or finger length. However, they still won't have a fingernail (unless a fingernail was present before the surgical intervention).

This surgery involves removing just the bone from the toe and placing it in the finger. Typically, a small wire temporarily holds the position while it heals for a few

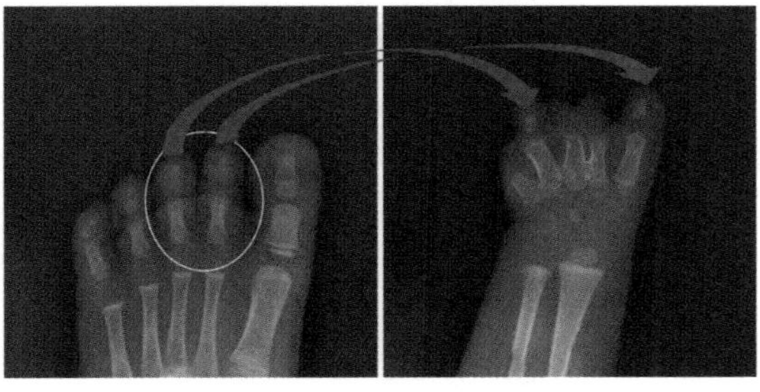

Figure 6-4: A partial toe bone-to-hand transfer. The hand x-ray (right) with added bones. The foot x-ray (left) after toe bones are moved; the soft parts of the toes remain.

weeks under a cast. In some surgeries, the toe bone may not grow well in this new location, and the surgery can be less successful.

Partial toe bone transfer surgery tends to be more successful in younger children under the age of 3. If the new bone does fit right in and starts growing, it can even be made longer by some of the lengthening techniques described above. If it doesn't work, the transplanted toe bone will simply dissolve, leaving the nubbin the same although possibly firmer. Once the phalanx bone is removed from the toe, the toe will be wigglier, sometimes shorter and less developed, but children will walk and run as expected.

In the future, interventions may include using man-made or laboratory-grown bone scaffold—an underlying material for bone growth, grafts, or the transfer of other small bones from somewhere else in the body, all of which could achieve the same goal for the hands without changing the toes at all. However, these new science advances would have to make bone that grows with the child, like their own bone would, and that discovery has not been made yet.

Finger Moving Surgeries on the Same Hand

Digits or fingers from the same hand can be rotated into a new position on the same hand. For example, children born without a thumb or a small thumb that can't bend can have the index finger rotated over into the thumb position and shortened so that it acts like a thumb. This surgery is called "pollicization" which means "making of a thumb." Other children may have a deep space or cleft in the middle of the hand, and fingers can be moved to close that space or make more room between the thumb and index finger to improve pinch. Rotated fingers keep their own arteries and nerves as they move into the new place. Those fingers can only move as far as their arteries and nerves allow.

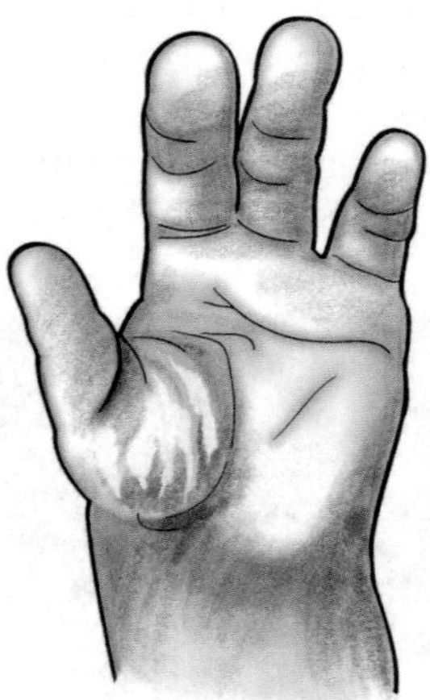

Figure 6-5: Pollicization is a surgery that rotates and shortens the index finger to the right size and position to work like a thumb.

Entire Toe Transfers

Children born with digit development that they can't move for any sort of functionality can have 1, 2, or even all their toes moved up to their hand. This toe transfer surgery has been done successfully by microsurgeons for decades. Preoperative testing is required to make sure the hand has enough arteries, tendons, ligaments, veins, and muscles to keep the transplanted toe healthy and functional in its new location. Typically, a child needs wrist bones and hand bones (metacarpals) to have this procedure. After surgery, the child will benefit from therapy and training to learn how to use their new digits.

Toe transfer surgery includes the fascinating science of microsurgery: studying exactly the anatomy of an area, muscle, organ, or limb of the body and what keeps that area connected to the rest of us. Then, using a microscope, surgeons carefully remove that part from one's own body, preserving the arteries, veins, nerves, tendons, muscles, and joints. Then, they reattach it to another part of the body, hooking it up to local sources of blood, nerve, veins, bone, and muscle in that new location. Muscles from the back and leg that are easy to live without can be transferred to various parts of the body depending on what is needed. It is a kind of transplant on the same child. This can be done with whole toes moved up to the hand to act like a finger.

Microsurgery and the ability to move a digit from one part of the body to another has been a significant leap in the field of congenital hand surgery and gives children a digit that can feel, touch, grab, bend, and nearly function as a finger. It has given some children functions they would not have otherwise had. The appearance after surgery will be similar to but not exactly like a finger, as toes are shorter and rounder in the end. Children who have toes transferred seem to do better when it's the second or third toe, although the big toe can be used as well. Children with these surgeries can walk and run and play as expected. Toe and foot alignment may not always be predictable as the child grows over time, and a visible difference to the foot is possible.

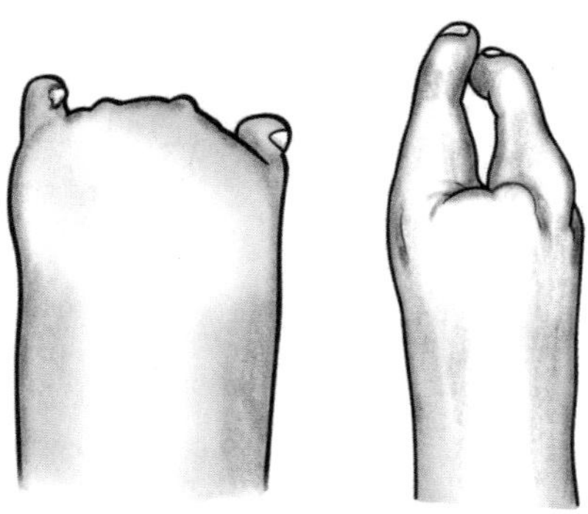

Figure 6-6: A complete toe-to-hand transfer, leaving the foot without those toes.

Typically, this surgery is done with children who have congenital hand differences by about 3 years of age. Similar to our language learning analogy, completing these surgical interventions earlier will help the child adapt to the new language earlier—these surgeries will change how the child will learn to pinch and grasp objects. While it is not impossible to have these surgeries when children are older, you will be asking the child to learn a new way to use their hands and forget the old way that they knew. Because of this, these surgeries are not typically done on older children/teens/adults.

Entire toe transfers may be recommended, however, for children, teens, and adults who have had an amputation later in their lives. Surgeons work to create a similar way of functioning that the child/teen/adult had prior to the acquired amputation.

Straightening Surgeries

When fingers or arms are partially formed, for example from amniotic bands around them, they can change shape. When it comes to curvatures, it's important to assess how form and function work together. Sometimes having a straight finger can help with function, but sometimes it might not. Surgeons assess if a child has a digit and thumb that can meet each other to pinch. For example, if the child has a pinky and thumb that bend toward each other, it might be easier to pinch because of the curvatures. Straightening these fingers may prevent the functional pinch.

Surgeries to straighten a bone or create more bend for greater function are typically achieved by breaking the bone, resetting it, and allowing it to heal in a new position. This may require a z-plasty or skin graft as well. Typically, the bone is held in place with temporary pins or wires (imagine an earring post coming outside

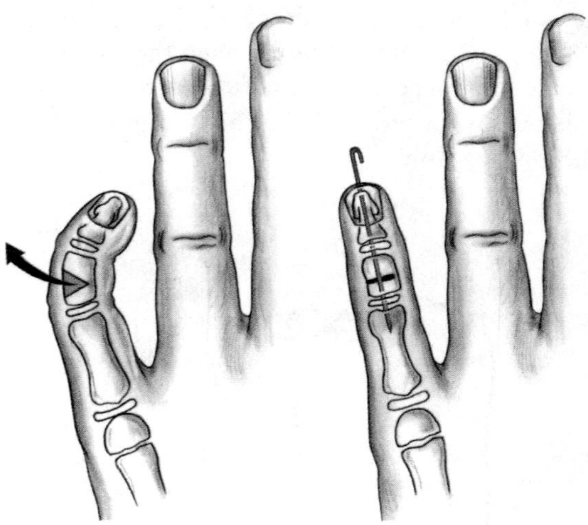

Figure 6-7: Bone straightening surgery with a temporary wire or pin that is inserted into the bone from outside the skin but is hidden from the child under the bandage or cast. The pin is smooth and can be easily removed in the doctor's office along with the cast/dressings after the skin and bone heal.

the finger). A cast or splint will be over the wire. As the bone heals from the resetting, the thin wires can be removed easily by sliding them out. The space from where the wires were will fill in with new bone quickly.

Metallic plates and screws are used in cases where the bone takes longer to heal. These small plates and screws are placed under the skin, so there is no need to have them removed, even after the bone has healed. If the hardware is irritating to the patient, it can be removed with another surgery. As these are surgeries that can change how the child's hand will function, the same age range recommendation of about 3 years old and under generally applies. However, these types of surgeries may be requested by an older child who wants them for specific reasons. In that case, they are offered only if the child will actively engage in the rehabilitation and the new form and function of their own hand.

REGENERATIVE SCIENCE

At one point, we were all just a few cells. Getting a few cells from umbilical cord blood or stem cells to turn into an arm or a finger may be possible someday. There are even science discoveries happening now where whole organs can be grown from a single kind of cell. Won't it be amazing when unique cells can be grown in a lab and then perhaps 3D-printed into the shape of a bladder or an esophagus?

While growing some replacement parts may be part of the future, growing an arm presents more of a challenge. The arm truly starts at the spinal cord and at the heart. There are artery, vein, and lymph cells; tendon, muscle, and ligament cells; bone, nail, cartilage, and synovial joint lining cells; and a myriad of other types of unique cells that work in concert to create the arm and hand. It's unlikely that scientists will be able to print or grow a part of a hand—or a full hand—and attach it successfully to a partially formed arm. Scientists first need to understand the cellular pattern of how limbs grow in the first place.

But will it be possible one day in the future? Scientists are learning about the potential of regenerative science in many different ways. There are salamanders, lizards, and even some fish that can regrow a tail when you remove it. Nearly a century or more of research has focused on understanding how those animals can regrow lost limbs. We know we all start out with those few "everything cells" or stem cells, which eventually become unique, such as cells that make up a hand. Figuring out the messaging that tells those cells how to become unique is called stem cell research. There's much we just don't know about how it all works, but as scientists consider studying how bodies form and develop in the womb, we can hope that one day regenerative science will be a viable treatment.

TRANSPLANT MEDICINE

Organ transplants from a donor child are possible today, but transplants for limb differences involve a larger set of problems. The biggest issue remains finding effective ways to prevent the receiving body from rejecting the parts of the donor. Transplant recipients often take steroids and immune system suppressing drugs for their whole lifetime, medications that can put a child's growth and health at risk.

We know that children who also have kidney or liver transplants are ideal candidates for hand transplants because they already take those medicines. In 2015, a child who was a kidney transplant recipient received 2 new arms at once. Because of the major side effects of the transplant medications, healthy children with at least some fingers or hands that function are not good candidates for hand transplants. They just can't benefit as clearly as they could be harmed.

Some candidates might also be more ideal due to other circumstances. A child who always had an arm but lost it due to trauma or infection will have brain pathways that know how to use a transplanted hand and might be a better candidate. A child who never had fingers may be challenged learning how to use them, as it would require building out a whole section of the brain. Think of it again like learning a new language. If you learn Spanish or French when you are young, then that pathway is well developed. Trying to learn a new language past a certain age can be challenging and frustrating. Not impossible; however, these are considerations when reviewing options.

THE KEY TO SURGICAL SUCCESS IS YOU

Looking at surgical options can seem exciting and daunting. As a parent, you may be inundated by new vocabularies and medical questions. Ultimately, your hope is that your decisions can secure your child's quality of life. Without surgery, a person with a hand difference might use a prosthetic more or use 1 hand all the time. You can't predict the outcome of your decisions, but as a parent you can help give them the best chance for future success, whether that is surgery or not surgery.

DISCUSSION QUESTIONS

When you first heard about your child's hand difference, what was your hope for modern medicine?

Now that you've learned some of the surgical interventions that can help your child change the form and function of their hand differences, do you feel more empowered to make these decisions?

What treatments has your surgeon recommended?

What is more information you would like to know?

Surgery needs to have a goal in mind. Like traveling from New York to Florida, you have options for the best way to get there for your family. You may walk there or take a road trip, a train ride, or an airplane flight. All are possibilities, but what are the benefits and the goals of each one? To make decisions on where you are now and where you want to go, surgical interventions should have a clear goal. There are real risks with surgical interventions, although they are low, so your team has to make them thoughtfully. Ask your surgeon what surgeries are time dependent and when you need to make the decision. Does your child need to be 1, 3, 8, or 16 years old? What options will go away as a child ages?

The ability for your child to be happy and healthy is not given in the operating room or in a 3D-printed prosthetic. We encourage you to learn about the surgery options currently available for your child that could potentially change how their hand looks and works. Review the goals that your child has for themselves and review their current barriers for these goals. Make the decisions that are right for you and your family and work with your surgeon to answer as many questions as you can about the risk and benefits of the decisions.

CHAPTER SUMMARY

In this is chapter, we learned:

- That there are many surgical interventions to change the form and function of a child's hand difference
- That some surgical interventions are typically recommended at a younger age
- That surgical decisions may need to be made by parents without the contribution of the child themselves. As the child ages, be sure to discuss with them as developmentally appropriate.
- That the more you know and the more you understand, the more likely the surgical interventions are to meet your expectations
- To bring lots of questions to the people who are most likely to know the answers

Chapter 7

Hand Prosthesis: Exploring Tools

In this Chapter

IN THIS CHAPTER, WE WILL LEARN:

- The basic options for prostheses
- How to explore prostheses
- Basic terms for prostheses

The term "prosthetics" refers to the profession of evaluation, fabrication, and fitting of prostheses. A prosthesis is the name of the device itself. The term "prosthetic" can be used as an adjective describing the type of artificial device—such as "prosthetic hands" or a "prosthetic nose." Prostheses are tools that may or may not be beneficial for your child and are always options for children throughout their life course. The choice is individual: there are many people who have and use prostheses, many who have never used them, and others who tried them and decided they did not want to use them. There is wide variation. Know that when making this decision, you and your child will have lots of time and many options to choose from when working with your prosthetist.

By exploring various types of devices, you can better understand how they work and explore terminology. As you learn more about all available options, you will feel empowered to make choices best for your family.

INTRODUCTION TO PROSTHETICS: PROSTHESES ARE TOOLS

A prosthesis is a tool that can help a person perform the tasks they need or want to do. A prosthesis is not a substitute for a missing hand or arm. The prosthesis doesn't affect whether your child will participate in an activity; it simply changes the way in which they will do it. It's merely a different way for the child to perform a task.

The hand and arm are incredibly intricate parts of the body, capable of performing both needlepoint and weightlifting. Today, prostheses come in a wide range of options, from prosthetic fingers that extend beyond existing nubs to whole hands and arms with fine motor skill motion. Some prostheses provide a way to grip or push while others feature muscle sensors to facilitate prosthetic finger or wrist movement. Prosthetic technology has developed devices to meet the needs of the full range of users, from full prosthetic arms with shoulder, elbow, wrist and finger joints all the way to partial hands/partial fingers.

The health care professional who designs and fits your child's device is called a prosthetist. Their role is to work with you and your child to provide the best technology and type of device based on the activities your child enjoys or tasks they want to accomplish and the barriers they are currently facing. How your child uses a device will be something the prosthetist will work with over time. Some individuals with upper limb differences choose to always wear their devices, while others choose to wear them only for specific activities. Still, some opt to not wear or use a prosthetic device at all. You and your child have all of these options.

Prostheses are not required. Whether or not you or your child chooses a device at all is truly dependent on your child's and your family's preferences. Many children can be successful without them, while others may find that challenging tasks are easier to complete with them. Some children may want a prosthesis to change or hide their appearance, while others do not like the way a prosthesis looks. You will want to ensure you have discussions with your child at each phase of development to see if the current device is helpful and useful or what other devices may be more beneficial.

If you are interested, you can follow prosthetic technology updates, reviews from other consumers, or prosthetic company representatives to keep up with current trends or devices that may be available for your child. Be sure to have conversations with your health care providers to understand their recommendations as well as with insurance companies to be aware of out-of-pocket prosthetic device costs and maintenance.

Know that there are lots of opinions about using or not using a prosthesis. Consider suggestions from your medical team and community and ultimately make the decision that is most beneficial for and supports your child. Remember, too, that your child will outgrow a prosthesis just as they outgrow their shoes.

A child must also be able to understand that a prosthesis is not a "new hand." Children believe in magic—up until around 6 to 7 years of age. Children may reject a prosthesis that does not meet the expectation of a real hand. Studies have shown that many children will dutifully wear their prosthesis for their parents and for doctor appointments, but will take it off in the car on the way home. A prosthesis is a big investment both in time and money and, just as surgery, has to have a particular goal. Until your child needs the prosthesis to accomplish a particular goal, they may not be ready for a prosthesis. Be sure to keep an ongoing conversation and check in about goals and needs.

DISCUSSION QUESTIONS

Are you considering how a device might benefit your child?

What 3 activities or roles in your child's life do they want a prosthesis to facilitate?

How could these be solved by a prosthesis?

THE ROLE OF THE PROSTHETIST

People explore prostheses at all stages of development. Some children may have their first device at 6 months old, particularly if it can help facilitate crawling, although research does indicate that a device at this age is not necessary, and children can coordinate crawling and balance without them. Others may have their first devices in their 40s looking to help facilitate a new hobby like painting or woodworking.

If you decide to explore prostheses, you will need a referral from your medical staff—usually your general practitioner, physical therapist, or hand surgeon. With a referral, you and your child will meet with the prosthetist, a medical professional with a master's level education and training in assessing and developing prosthetic systems for your child. Your prosthetist will ask your child and your family about the goals you want to achieve and barriers you are facing.

Your prosthetist will be your resource in exploring the variety of device options to meet the goals that you discussed. You and your child will continue to work with a prosthetist as your child grows and their needs change. Your prosthetist will make adjustments, facilitate repairs and replacements, and explore additional devices as needed.

TYPES OF PROSTHESES

The prosthesis can come with many different adjustable and customizable parts. Selecting these features will be part of the conversations you have with your prosthetist as they build a device system for your child. There are several systems of prostheses that relate to how the device is powered, the connection points and features, and the types of terminal ends available for that specific system. Each system has its own customizable components; however, some may not as easily be able to switch parts from different prosthetic systems. Your child may have multiple prostheses for multiple actions.

Static or Passive Devices

Static devices (or sometimes called passive devices) do not have moving components. If your child is young, a prosthetist might recommend a passive hand prosthesis designed to look lifelike without moving parts. For younger children like toddlers, a passive hand may be useful for balance or 2-handed grip activities such as crawling, holding a paper on the table while writing, or catching a beach ball.

As your child grows, you will have a better sense of your child's hand functionality, adaptability, and sense of self, which will be important as you explore other options. If a passive device doesn't meet all their needs, you can next explore more complex devices with moving parts or even robotic technology.

Static devices can also be made as tools for a specific activity. For example, your child might have a lightweight sports arm to help with balance or a static hand for dancing. Other options can include a yoga arm that has a flattened terminal device to facilitate actions such as push-ups, downward dog poses, or handstands. Static devices can have attachments to facilitate hanging or holding onto trapezes, pull-up bars, or gymnastics bars. Some devices can even have sports equipment attached to the device such as a mitt, a net, or a cupped shape designed to hold various balls. Even without moving parts, a static device provides functionality and can be the perfect tool for a number of jobs.

Static devices can serve a cosmetic function, which means that the arm's design and function is to look like an expected arm and hand. Some devices have fingernails that can be painted. Often there will be a realistic hand component with the fingers in a resting hand position with the fingers slightly cupped and the thumb resting in line with the wrist. Imagine the position your hands would take when you are standing and they are relaxed at your side. Static arms can serve several functions and may meet your child's needs.

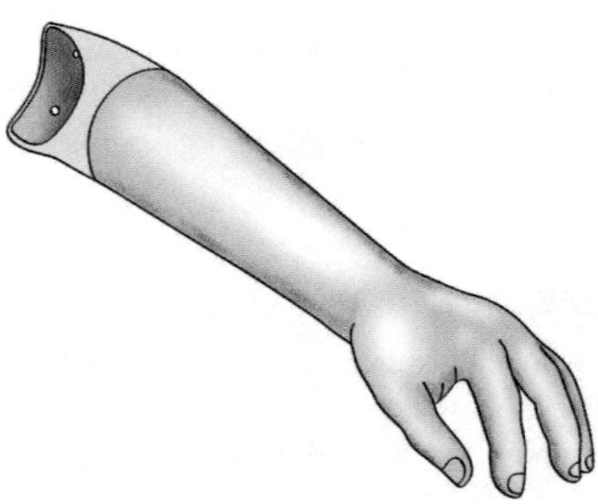

Figure 7-1: A static prosthetic upper limb.

Body-Powered Devices

Body-powered devices are prostheses that have moving pieces powered by the user's own body. Their functionality is dependent on working the device with the body, usually by protracting (pushing forward) or retracting (pulling back) the shoulder. This type of prosthesis might have a terminal device that resembles a hand, a hook, or another shape that can open and close based on the user moving their arm or shoulder.

To make a body-powered device work with a hook, for example, the user wears the socket with a shoulder harness that can be worn under or over clothing. Using shoulder motions, the user opens the hook by pushing the shoulder forward and can close the hook by pulling the shoulder back.

Body-powered devices can also include moving pieces that require an external force to operate. The user might use their other hand to position the fingers and/or wrist on their prosthetic hand.

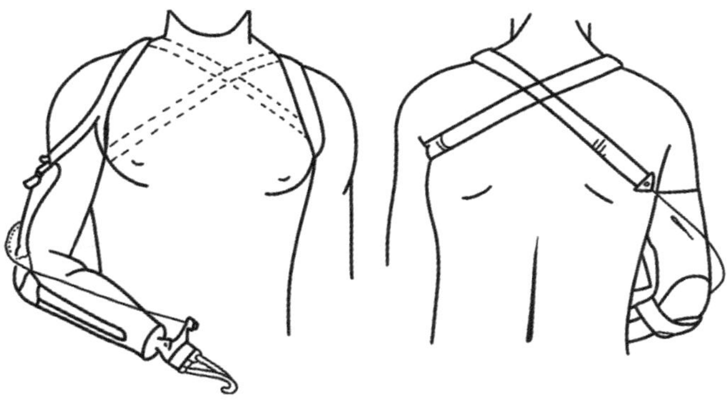

Figure 7-2: A body-powered device with harness.

Myoelectric Devices

A myoelectric prosthesis is operated by the electric signals coming from the wearer's own muscles. These devices feature robotic hands and may look very futuristic, with some users identifying with the bionic nature of their prosthesis. The device works with muscles present in the hand, forearm, or upper limb. Myoelectric devices allow the user to wear multifunction hands—this means it gives users the opportunity to have different "grips" or grip patterns with their bionic hand or end terminal device. This is attractive to many users as they may want more specific and fine motor functionality than the basic "open/close" options of body-powered devices.

Presently, there are 2 versions of myoelectric devices: one/two site myoelectric and pattern recognition. Both versions require placing electrodes within the user's socket to "read" muscle movement. As muscles in the residual limb contract, electrical impulses are read by the electrodes in the prosthetic device. The electrodes relay that information to the bionic hand to allow the user to create multiple grips, each providing different functionality for the wearer. Your clinician will be able to share the intricacies with you between these 2 methods and provide you with the best path depending on what your child wants to do and needs to do.

It takes training and practice working with health care professionals for these movements to feel easy and intuitive. Users are learning a new language as they relearn how they interact with their environment. Be mindful of the frustration tolerance of your child at the time when exploring devices. It is OK to pause learning and pick it back up later if other events are happening in your child's life taking up time and energy. It is important to be mindful of the other activities and events happening in your child's life when scheduling therapy sessions for a new device. Big things like starting a new school, major exams, or moving may not be the best times to begin learning a new device. Be sure to have open dialogue with your child.

Myoelectric devices have electric power needs and require charging and maintenance for moving parts. Some users have even reported that the robotic movements make electronic sounds that can be fairly loud. Depending on the context of how and where the user is wearing the device, noise from the hand or finger action might not always be welcome, such as when hearing electronic movements in class, at religious events, or even at home.

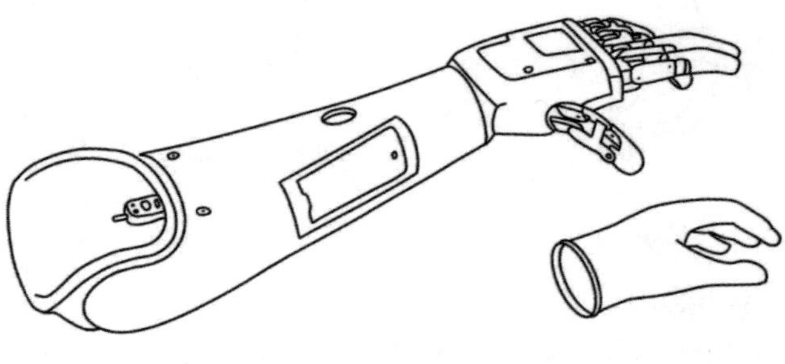

Figure 7-3: A myoelectric prosthesis.

DISCUSSION QUESTIONS

What are your thoughts on prostheses?

What would you like the prosthesis to allow your child to do that they can't do as easily now?

Think about how you might talk to your child about what a prosthesis might mean to them. What questions would you ask?

3D-PRINTED TECHNOLOGY

Some devices can include 3D-printed hand- or finger-like components, allowing wearers to use the movement of their wrist or elbow to flex and extend the fingers. 3D-printed devices are new and can be exciting. Many professional clinics are beginning to experiment with 3D-printed designs; however, this is still an emerging field. As technology and research advance in the prosthetic world, it is very likely 3D printing is going to be something that emerges within it.

Some 3D-printed devices are created by clubs or organizations for school groups that may have limited research or knowledge on prosthesis, user interfaces, body anatomy, or body mechanics. The components can be made at home affordably, which can make them attractive.

Plastics for 3D-printed objects may not be durable, and the pieces can be small and fragile. 3D-printed hands also can be cosmetic and quite colorful and may be a fun way to introduce prostheses to children. If you are considering exploring 3D-printed devices, set up appropriate expectations for the device depending on where the device was created and the technology used behind it.

DEVICE FEATURES

Different device systems will give your child various things. Not all device systems are created the same or can perform the same function. Let's explore some features when considering device systems.

Sensory feedback is the user receiving information about the object they want to interact with. A person can pick up, say, a water glass, and when using a typically developed hand, they can easily adjust the amount of force they use to pick up a water glass between a full water glass (using more strength) or an empty water glass (using less strength). Their brains and hands have calibrated this to be effective in their gripping, and they can feel the weight of the glass when first picking it up (this is sensory feedback). When a person has a limb difference, they interact with objects with their limb-different hands, adjusting their bodies as needed to accommodate the weight of the glass in their adaptive strategies, because they can get the sensory feedback on their bare skin.

When this residual limb is placed into a prosthesis, aspects of this sensory feedback are altered since this portion of the hand is covered. This is an important aspect to consider to both set up expectations for current prosthetic technology and help facilitate conversations with your prosthetist.

Cosmesis means the appearance of the hand. Does the wearer typically like the way the hand looks, and is this easily accepted into social climates? Having a prosthesis that both looks and functions in a way that works best for your child is important. Some people may really like the look of a hook or may really like the look of a robotic-looking hand. Others want their hands to resemble a typically developed hand. All of these are valid options. Celebrate the option your child wants.

Weight refers to the actual weight of the device. Myoelectric devices are heavy, as they have moving portions and need to have electrical components in the device itself, whereas a passive hand does not have these aspects and will be lighter in weight. This is important to consider as the wearer will need to develop the tolerance, strength, and endurance to wear devices for longer periods of time and will likely work with a therapist to develop a wear schedule so as not to burn out the arm from immediate all-day use.

Durability is the device's ability to withstand everyday use or even use on tougher activities. Body-powered hooks are more durable than myoelectric hands, as the myoelectric hands have multiple moving parts. Myoelectric hands are not ideal for lifting weights or carrying heavy objects. Often, fingers break or the device needs repairs more frequently in engaging in these types of activities, whereas more passive devices that are designed for weightlifting may be better fits for these activities.

DECIDING WHAT'S RIGHT FOR YOU AND YOUR CHILD

Be sure to have multiple conversations with health care professionals, your child, your family, and your insurance company to determine if and what type of prosthetic systems would be beneficial for your child. Your child can trial multiple devices and find what works best for them. Have conversations with your child to determine their needs and how various devices could potentially fit those needs. Be open to changing the idea of what the prosthetic device will be. Sometimes people may want a particular type of device but find that another system entirely is better for achieving the goal they desire.

Keep in mind that at this point in technology we are unable to both replace a hand in appearance and have it work and function as a hand does. This can be hard for children and their families to accept. If you or your child need more support or are facing major barriers, please talk through these themes with your health care providers and see what support they can provide.

PROSTHESIS SELECTION IS A JOURNEY

Prosthetics is a rapidly growing and developing field with new technological advancements. The options for prostheses are available for the full duration of your child's life. Your child may be interested when they are younger, may choose to use them, then not use them, or explore different options. It is all a fluid journey, and prosthetics as a field is here for your child whenever (and if ever) your child finds it useful. Many successful adults have found their devices helpful, and many other successful adults chose not to use them; it is all dependent on what your child wants and finds useful.

DISCUSSION QUESTIONS

What are your and your child's expectations and hopes for a prosthesis?

How can those guide you and your child while learning about and exploring prosthetic options?

Who are the people and organizations you are partnering with to develop a prosthetic system? What is their background, and how does this impact your expectations for the device?

CHAPTER SUMMARY

In this chapter, we learned:

- That there are different prosthetic systems for your child, and each system has various features and goals
- That you can work with a prosthetist to design devices that work best for your child
- That prostheses are tools to help your child do the things they want and need to do. It's OK if your child does or does not choose to explore prostheses.
- That you can work with your child to explore prostheses at any point in their life course

Chapter 8

Hand Therapy: Adaptations and Functional Training

In this Chapter

IN THIS CHAPTER, WE WILL LEARN:

- About occupational, physical, and mental health therapists and their unique scope of practice and training
- About the therapeutic process
- About adaptive products, tools, and training

Therapeutic interventions can help address strength and range of motion and develop adaptive strategies and coping mechanisms for people to engage in activities they need to do and want to do. There are several types of therapists with whom your child can work. They will provide expertise in specific areas depending on clinical and training background. It is important to keep in mind that a good relationship with your child's therapist is important. If your child is not connecting with their therapist, you can request to change. Therapists typically need a referral from a general practitioner, a hand surgeon, or school evaluations and assessments.

TYPES OF THERAPIES

Mental health therapists, physical therapists, and occupational therapists will all most likely be part of your care team at some point. They can provide an array of therapies to help you and your child feel confident and adjusted and facilitate engagement in the activities your child needs and wants to do. Each provider will establish goals with your child and your family and will monitor progress toward those goals.

Mental health therapists are trained in developmental psychology and therapeutic interventions to best support and address the psychological and psychosocial health of children and/or families. They may have tools and strategies to address a variety of mental health conditions such as depression and anxiety, and they may help address restructuring belief systems of children with differences/disabilities. (Be open to the need for a mental health professional for your own or other family members' needs as well.)

Physical therapists (PTs) work to improve strength and movement as your child grows and develops. They may advise, perform, or recommend exercises to stretch, strengthen, or rehabilitate arms and hands after surgery.

Occupational therapists (OTs) can work with your child to engage in functional activities that your child needs to do and wants to do throughout their day. They can work on adapting objects and tools or devise adaptive strategies for children to complete activities such as dressing, toileting, feeding, writing, playing musical instruments, playing sports, and playing in general. OTs can also be seen for rehabilitation after surgery.

These services are available in the public school setting depending on whether your child qualifies for services under current federal policies.

Each therapist will have their own unique set of training and background. They may have a specialty in pediatrics or in hand-related therapies. Therapists may practice specific forms of therapy, and this is determined by the setting they work in, or they may be able to employ various types of therapeutic interventions. Each therapist achieved the highest level of education required at the time of their graduation from training programs. This accounts for various types of degrees. Some therapists who were trained in the 1980s and 1990s have bachelor's degrees in their field, as master's programs or doctorate programs were unavailable, whereas students training today may be required to have master's or doctorate degrees. Regardless of the degree type, each therapist is trained and has experience to assist you and your child. Each therapist was required to sit for national board exams to be allowed to practice nationally and will have applied for a license to practice in your state. Each year, all these therapists are required to complete continuing education credits in their area of therapy through approved education institutions to ensure they stay informed on current trends and new practices. Have conversations with your therapist about their background and training in your child's specific needs. Ask what professional organizations they belong to. This can ensure that your child has a good fit with their therapist.

DISCUSSION QUESTIONS

What are 3 of your child's strengths?

Is there anything your child wants to do but is having a tough time doing?

Where do you think these barriers come from? Are they physical, social, or emotional?

Do you have an idea about how to make an activity easier for your child? Brainstorm with your therapists about adapting household items, musical instruments, sports equipment, and other things to make it easier for your child to participate.

THE THERAPEUTIC PROCESS

You will likely need a referral from your primary physician for therapy and will be recommended to a therapist or clinic for services. The initial intake appointment will likely be a longer appointment. During this visit, the therapist will ask you and your child several questions and may take measurements to get a good picture of where your child is presently, as well as identify strengths and barriers. They will also talk with you and your child about the things your child wants to do. Your therapist will develop goals based on the findings in the initial intake and will develop a treatment plan. This plan will outline therapy session lengths (likely 30 minutes to 1 hour) and session frequency (1 to 7 days a week). They will also provide a treatment timeline to achieve these goals, such as over 4 sessions or by 3 months.

Sometimes goals are addressed and met in the initial intake, such as creating or fitting a splint or developing an exercise program. Other times therapy will progress over the course of several weeks. At each therapy session, your therapist will have developed activities for your child to complete that will help them progress toward their goals. At any point goals can be edited, canceled, or added depending on your child's needs.

During the session, your therapist will make notes on your child's progress and will make adjustments to therapy sessions to appropriately challenge your child. At the end of every session, your therapist will document progress in their notes and will report on progress toward goals. If the goals are achieved early and no more needs are identified, it is likely that your child will be discharged from therapy early with a home maintenance program. Therapists can also extend the timeline if they believe your child would benefit from additional sessions.

Therapy costs may or may not be reimbursed by insurance companies. Be mindful of in-network and out-of-network providers and work with your insurance company to understand costs.

THERAPEUTICS WITH PROSTHESIS

If a child is getting a new prosthesis, it will likely come with a set of OT sessions to help teach the child how to use their hand and explore device features. Often prostheses are heavy. This additional weight to the end of the arm may cause the child's arm to fatigue more quickly. OTs will work with you and your child to develop goals and assess barriers so your child can engage in all the activities they care about and feel empowered to use their prosthesis.

Therapeutic plans help strengthen the child's arm to be able to tolerate longer periods of time using the arm before fatigue sets in. Therapy can explore functional activities like zipping up jackets while using the prosthetic device or can include exercises to practice repetition of fine motor activities like picking up and releasing small blocks.

Just as important as a good socket fit, having the knowledge to use the prosthesis as a tool will enhance your child's ability to use the device and find it useful.

HAND DOMINANCE

Discussions of hand dominance are uniquely relevant to early school and sports activities such as writing or throwing. Children will explore and interact with objects in their environment with the limbs they have. Depending on the form and function of their limb difference, they may use the limb with a hand difference a lot, use it as a helper or assist hand, or use it as the primary hand. Children around the age of 5 tend to choose hand dominance, using their dominant hand to initiate interacting with objects. Children with hand differences tend to use their unaffected hand as their dominant hand only because it can be more functional. If both hands are limb-different, they'll tend to make the lesser-affected hand their dominant hand.

You may see a child with a right-sided limb difference use their left hand as their dominant hand but kick balls with their right foot. You may see children who are ambidextrous and use both hands. Allow the child to develop hand dominance most natural to them. If you would like extra support, you can ask your pediatrician for an OT referral prescription. OTs can specialize in hand therapy and handwriting and will develop strategies for your child.

ADAPTING AND ADJUSTING

"If there is a will, there is a way." There will be a way your child can complete the activities they need to do and want to do. There are many solutions! Children are exceptionally creative and often discover their own strategies.

There are hundreds of social media accounts and internet videos of children, teens, and adults engaging in 1-handed/no-handed activities. Try searching for "1-handed cooking" or "how to put up hair with 1 arm" or "how to fish with 1 hand"—you are likely to find multiple videos with various strategies. Modifications may require additional steps (eg, switching hands) or the use of other body parts like elbows, chest, hips, legs, knees, and feet. Some videos feature people with amputations or individuals with strokes—the condition or diagnosis is not important if the strategies are helpful. Your child may not adopt the suggested strategy; however, these videos may provide ideas for creating a method so your child can do the activity in question. You can request OT services for tools and strategies and develop a plan if your child is experiencing difficulty with tasks. The OT can teach new skills, break down steps, and give your child exercises to work on that will help develop the strength and range of motion needed for the task.

Many 1-handed products may replace common 2-handed products. Examples include 1-handed nail clippers, toothpaste dispensers, rocker knives, non-slip mats to stabilize a bowl while stirring, 1-handed salt and pepper grinders, 1-handed keyboards, and 1-handed envelope openers. You can find these products via web searches or on medical supply websites. Alternatively, you can improvise or create these products in your home. The difficulty with 1-handed products is that they are not common in all households. A child may really find it beneficial to use a 1-handed salt grinder at home; however, the restaurant may only have a 2-handed salt grinder. It is not feasible to purchase/build all new tools and to carry the products around for possible use. Some tools seem like they would be beneficial but then turn out not to be. Be mindful of the tools that your child will benefit from, and try out different things!

You may or may not work with a therapist or you may work with all these therapists. These are resources for you and your child to use at any point in their life course. You may find a great combination of surgery, prosthetics, and therapeutic interventions, you may choose 1 intervention, or you may use some at different points as your child grows up. These are all tools and resources for your child to do all the things they need and want to do.

CHAPTER SUMMARY

In this chapter, we learned:

- About the various types of therapists and their scope of practice
- About the therapeutic timeline
- To be empowered when making decisions about therapeutic services

Part III
Growing Up

Chapter 9

Stigma: Disability and Hand Differences

In this Chapter

IN THIS CHAPTER, WE WILL LEARN:

- How to explore childhood identity development and ways of communicating
- About various models of disability
- Important vocabulary to articulate your and your child's experience, such as stigma, ableism, internalized ableism, and microaggressions

Having a hand difference is common, but not common enough that everyone your child encounters has met someone else with a hand difference. This is still a new experience for some people, and there is a series of social frameworks and understanding of what it means to be different. There is a rich and vibrant history of disability advocacy. There are thousands of people who identify with disability who proudly fought for legislation and civil rights protection in beautiful and creative ways. They led the longest federal government building sit-in, lasting 28 days at the US Department of Health, Education, and Welfare in San Francisco in April 1977. Students at Gallaudet University, for students who identify as Deaf and hard of hearing, protested their university's failure to select a Deaf person as president of the university. Activists climbed the US Capitol stairs sans wheelchairs to encourage the passing of the Americans with Disabilities Act (ADA). In this chapter, we will review the science and models developed to understand and articulate the disabled experience, why culture shifts are important, and how you and your child can advocate for yourselves.

LEGAL DEFINITIONS OF DISABILITY

Disability is the term selected by disability rights activist leaders like Judy Heumann, Ed Roberts, Justin Dart, Fusako Tanida, and Brad Lomax in 1990 with the passing of the ADA and Section 504 of the Rehabilitation Act of 1973. Disability is a legal term, as defined by the ADA and Rehabilitation Act: "An individual with a disability is a person who has a physical or mental impairment that substantially limits one or more major life activities, has a record of such impairment or is regarded as having such an impairment."

This definition covers people with limb differences, as their daily activities are impacted by their limb difference. Even though they are adaptable and may have different strategies, the limb difference does impact the way they do their tasks. They are also legally regarded as having a disability, which covers them as well.

Section 504 of the Rehabilitation Act of 1973 protects individuals with disabilities from discrimination in any federally funded or related programs and activities. This is the piece of legislation that will support students in the classroom setting.

The ADA is a significant piece of legislation that provides civil rights protections to individuals with disabilities in various forms of public life, such as accommodations, transportation, government services, and communications. This is the piece of legislation that ensures public buildings and transportation provide reasonable accommodations to support people with disabilities in their employment.

The term "disability" is not necessarily a medical term; there is no diagnosis of "disability." Disability is a self-identifying umbrella term where an individual may have a specific diagnosis that will fall within the legal term of disability. For example, a child may have the medical diagnosis of TAR syndrome, and TAR is covered legally by disability laws. Sometimes limb differences have a specific diagnostic term, and sometimes terms will change as we continue to research and better understand development. Oftentimes in health care you may come across terms such as "impairments" or the phrase "functional impairments." These are limitations that a person is experiencing as a result of their condition. Impairment is a term regularly used in medical literature.

LET'S TALK ABOUT STIGMA

Stigma is the social perception of something that is unwanted. There is a social expectation for humans to look and function in a specific way. When people do not fit this idea, they are faced with social limitations. In recent years, there have been social and cultural shifts that are beginning to broaden the definition of expected human variation in American society. Stigma is a negative reaction to people who are different from what society expects. Your emotions may be driven by these reactions to your child. Like any other worry or fear, once you understand why it is happening, you can overcome it.

Some people may use the term "disability" when talking about your child's hand difference. It may make you cringe at such a loaded term. Let's explore why.

In the United States today, disability is not typically a positive attribute. We are better today than, say, in 1920 when people with disabilities were placed in institutions. Hopefully, attitudes will continue to improve in the coming years due to greater acceptance of all sorts of differences. Though our society still has many areas in which to grow in supporting individuals with physical differences, we work with what we have today. There are over 300 million people in the United States, each unique in appearance and how they function. Yet, this is not represented in our media outlets. This is true for roughly 25% of Americans, or over 80 million people, who have a physical, mental, or emotional disability. This lack of representation and awareness may make your child feel like a novelty to others, and some may have a tough time understanding their experience.

Many parents may never have been introduced to these themes and concepts. Perhaps, before they were parenting a child with a hand difference, they assumed hand differences to be a "disability" or a "bad thing." These thoughts are usually accompanied with negative feelings. For example, because society has taught them to view a child with hand differences as "less than perfect," parents may feel shame, guilt, or embarrassment. As a way to combat this shame, parents may proclaim that *their* child does not have a disability. However, this messaging threatens the pride of the disability culture because it reinforces that disability is a thing to be ashamed of and that their child is not a part of that shameful thing. This is because of prevailing values in the society we were raised in and internalizing these thoughts without processing or understanding them.

These negative emotions are the product of a world where many people have been raised to expect that people come in a specific body type. "Ableism" is the term for discrimination based on how someone functions or appears. It operates much as do other "-isms," under which an entire group is thought less capable or inferior in any number of ways and subject to limitations and barriers. Many of these attitudes are based on a lack of understanding and fear of those of us who are somehow different. A child with a congenital limb difference may challenge some people to see that child as a whole and complete person.

DISCUSSION QUESTIONS

What does ableism mean to you?

What does disability mean to you?

What are the messages you receive from society and culture about people with physical differences?

How has the world you grew up in shaped your perspective?

THE SCIENCE OF GRIEF

Let's unpack grief and how it relates to the stigma of being a part of a minority group. Social values in the United States have an emphasis on independence or the ability to care for oneself. Having a child with a hand difference challenges our idea of what independence is. Therefore, various emotions of loss and feelings of grief can be generated.

What is grief? In 1969, psychiatrist Elisabeth Kübler-Ross outlined 5 stages of grief in her book *On Death and Dying*: denial, anger, bargaining, depression, and acceptance. Five stages occur in dealing with any situation that involves mourning a loss, whether it is the loss of a loved one or the expectation of a different future. In 1975, pediatric researchers at Case Western Reserve University School of Medicine expanded on this theory and developed a hypothetical model for parents who have a child with a congenital difference. The model is divided into 2 parts—reactive roles and active roles. Reactive roles are those in which parents are reacting to the information of a congenital difference. The active roles show how parents can initiate and take responsibility for their actions.

It is important to note that within both reactive and active parts, there are multiple stages of parent emotions. Not all parents will experience every emotion or expression of grief, nor is there a specific order through which everyone will experience them. This model helps provide language and context to help parents and others understand their reactions. In other words, it can help you understand what you're feeling and why you are feeling it. Some parents may stay in one phase for years, go back and forth between phases, or feel that they are simultaneously in more than one phase. It's all a part of the process, and parents should understand that they are not alone.

Reactive Roles Include:

Shock: Parents often experience huge shock when discovering a hand difference. Parents were not aware this was even possible and were completely unprepared for the news. Parents may not be able to think properly. They may have feelings of hopelessness and sadness. Parents may have a difficult time imagining a positive future for their child.

Denial: Parents may be in denial that their baby's hand is different and may pretend that the child has 2 hands and 10 fingers. Parents may not want to deal with the situation and may decide it is not real.

Sadness: The most common parent emotion reported in this research study was sadness. Parents reported crying frequently, even after a long time had passed.

Anger: Parents reported feeling angry at themselves, their child, their partner, or hospital staff. Some parents reported hating and blaming those around them for the event.

Anxiety: Parents reported feelings of anxiety and worry for their child's future, regardless of the reassurance provided by the people who support them. Some parents felt a lack of connection and attachment to their child due to fears and anxieties. This is something to be mindful of, as a lack of bonding with a child can impact the child's development. If you find that your or your child's loved ones are having a difficult time connecting with your child, seek out support from health care professionals or close friends.

Bargaining: Some parents may begin to suggest trades and bargain with a higher power to correct their child's hand difference, such as promising they will "never do X again" or offering to trade their own hands to give to their child.

Active Roles Include:

Adaptation: Parents begin to adapt by working to change perspective. Parents can begin to see their child as a whole child with a hand difference and acknowledge that their child has a hand that is different. Parents can begin to feel a connection with their child and see their strengths, which will help them embrace the congenital hand difference.

Reorganization: This is coming to the understanding that the hand difference is not anyone's fault and that the child will live a full and meaningful life. Parents can begin adapting activities, exploring problem solving, and supporting each other.

There is a transitioning process from reactive to active roles that may take a significant amount of emotional energy. Your child will likely be the one to lead you away from your initial reactions. You watch as your baby grows and explores their world. Suddenly you find yourself worrying more about babyproofing your home and protecting your bright and curious little one from harm than the hand difference. You will see your child's personality come through, and you will be amazed at how your child sees no obstacle if you will just get out of the way.

DISCUSSION QUESTIONS

Adjustment is not something that happens smoothly in a straight line. How has your adjustment been since day 1?

Draw a chart. Have you experienced any of the stages in the model of grief? If so, what are they, and what did they look like?

Has your partner or co-parent experienced any of the stages in the model of grief? If so, what were they, and what did they look like?

Have you and your partner/co-parent talked about feelings? What strategies do you have to start this conversation?

DISCUSSION QUESTIONS

When you think about the active roles, what are several things you can do now?

What are 3 things you can do to actively pursue adaptation and reorganization for you and your family?

To whom else can you model this behavior? Caregivers? Teachers?

MODELS OF DISABILITY

The disability identity helps connect all persons who live adaptive lives to a collective experience and community with a vibrant culture. Children with limb differences, no matter how big or how small, will navigate the world differently than people who do not have limb differences. This different experience is collectively shared among those who identify with the disability community. Let's explore the various models of disability. There are many theoretical models that help people understand and process disability within society and culture. The main ones discussed in this chapter are the social model of disability, the medical model of disability, and the interdependent model of disability.

Our limb-different children will be fully capable of doing the things they want to do and need to do. It's rather society and culture that have created a physical and social world with limited access. This concept is the basis of the **social model of disability**. For example, when some people see a person with a congenital hand difference, they assume they cannot type if they do not have all their fingers and thus cannot do computer-based tasks. The social model of disability views disability as a social construct, allowing that there is nothing inherently wrong with anyone's body, but rather problems are rooted in the social values inherent in a world where disability is unfavored. This theoretical model guarantees access to the individual by creating access in social and physical climates, such as fabricating adaptive tools and making modifications to a classroom.

Another model, the **medical model of disability**, describes a disability as something that can be remedied by medical or therapeutic intervention with the emphasis to bring the body as close to typically developing as possible. This theoretical model gives access to the individual by making modifications to their body through surgical or therapeutic interventions.

A newer model is the **interdependent model of disability**, which is the understanding that all humans are interdependent; no one is solely caring for oneself. People depend on others to grow food and create clothing. We are all providers and receivers of care necessary to address all our needs. Thus, communal care becomes important to people with disabilities since they may have a different set of needs—for example, standard architectural elements like stairs and doorknobs might not be usable by all. People with disabilities are not solely recipients of care; they are also contributors to the well-being of others. They may, through choices in life such as parenting or career, become an invaluable source of support, friendship, and creativity for others. This model grants access to an individual through understanding of individual needs and abilities to both receive and provide for others within the social climate.

People with hand differences will likely use, experience, and exist within all these models. There are times when medical interventions can provide a person with increased access, just as changing the way door handles are designed can provide more access for an individual. All the models of understanding disability may help the individual; no one model is better than others for understanding disability. When talking to service providers on receiving services or support for your child, be mindful of what theoretical model the person has been trained with and the scope of practice they operate under; this will flavor their perspective. Reflect on services offered or suggested for your child. Will they effectively reduce barriers and help provide access for your child?

DISCUSSION QUESTIONS

What are the messages you are receiving from others about your child's hand?

How are society and culture creating and/or limiting access for your child with a hand difference?

What are modifications or adaptations that you can make as a parent to create a more accessible environment for your child?

At this point in your journey, have medical interventions been suggested? What are the goals of these medical interventions for your child?

SELF-AWARENESS

Reflecting on theoretical models of disability and grief, it is important to consider the self-awareness development of your child as they grow up in a world with many messages. You can help guide them and develop an understanding of why messages are shared and what they can do to build positive messages about their hands.

Children begin to notice their hands as toddlers and may make comments such as, "Mommy, why is my hand different from yours?" They might even grow frustrated and say something like, "Daddy, I want a hand like yours." We know from research that 3-to-5-year-old children are aware that their hands look different and yet do not have difficulty with self-esteem. As a parent, you can view this sort of a comment for what it is—a toddler exploring the world around them and asking a simple question. Around the 6-to-8-year-old mark, children begin to look to the external environment for messages to develop their self-concept. They are trying to figure out how they view themselves and how they fit into the world around them. They become very aware of messaging and care about this messaging as they are developing who they are. Children of school age often navigate the stigmas and microaggressions, or subtle acts of discrimination, perpetuated by kids and adults around them. The messaging they are receiving about their hands may not always be positive.

While stigma is the negative assumptions of others, a microaggression is the action people take based on the stigmas they feel or believe. Think of a music teacher who believes "a child with a hand difference will not be able to play the piano." That's a stigma. A microaggression would be when the same teacher limits the opportunity for the child to play piano and only provides space for them to sing or play the tambourine. Children may be fearful and shy around each other at a most basic level, while others may turn that fear into action with taunts, making fun of the difference or rejecting the honest advances of a child who wants to be friendly.

Children at 8 years old are looking to develop their social hierarchies and determine where they fit in. They are upholding messages as to what is valued in society and rejecting the characteristics that are not valued. These messages are taught through their media outlets, books, TV shows, social media, movies, music videos, and advertising campaigns. Often, disability is not included in our inclusive campaigns, and children will pick up on the messages that disability is unfavored.

As a child with a difference receives these negative messages, they may begin to feel insecure. Research has shown that they enter a crisis, where they are receiving conflicting messages, such as the messages from family and friends like, "There is nothing wrong with you," and messages from strangers such as, "What's wrong with you?" Children may not want to return to school or be around the children who targeted or excluded them. Children this age lack the self-awareness skills to effectively cope with this crisis and may be left confused and asking for a quick solution.

They may begin asking to speak with medical professionals themselves; they may begin asking for a prosthetic hand or for surgery to "fix" their hand. You know they've just experienced the moment when they realized that their hand is different and that this difference means something to them socially. Children may experience the same type of shock and grief that parents experience when first learning of the hand difference.

Keep in mind that at this point in technology we are unable to both replace a hand in appearance and have it work and function as a typical hand does. This can be hard for children and their families to accept around the 8-year-old mark as they build their self-concepts. Be mindful that these realizations, thoughts, feelings, and messaging may be happening. Find ways to develop self-esteem, pride, and acceptance for the bodies we have and who we are.

Stigmas and microaggressions can threaten children's self-esteem during this time, and they may be vulnerable. Every child will feel and experience this differently. Some children will be impacted for an afternoon, and others may feel the impact for several years. Be mindful of your child's behaviors. Are you noticing any changes? Are they starting to hide their hand inside a sleeve or pockets more frequently? Are they increasingly withdrawn in public spaces or more resistant to do new activities with new people? Are they mentioning friends' names less or having fewer friend meetups? When you ask who the mean or trouble-maker kids are in class, can they identify them quickly and share more stories of them than stories of friends? This may be a good moment to begin conversations about your own experience as a child, or your own experiences of finding out about the hand difference. You want to model effective coping strategies for your child as they develop their own coping skills. If you feel your child has more of these withdrawn behaviors and it is starting to limit them from doing the things they used to love to do, reach out to your support network and/or medical care team. They can help brainstorm coping and self-esteem boosting strategies.

There is also a moment where microaggressions and bullying advance into larger acts of discrimination. If bullying ever grows to an intensity that your child feels too isolated or uncomfortable to engage in school or playground activities, this is important to bring up to your school administration. Your child has the legal right under the ADA and 504 to engage in school and the activities they want and need to do. These laws protect your child from discrimination and may support necessary changes in your child's school setting.

The crisis at 6 to 8 years of age varies from child to child in impact and duration. Some children may feel it for an afternoon and find ways to resolve it quickly. Others can show lasting effects that may need a lot of time and energy to resolve. All children with hand differences will experience these difficulties from time to time, just as we all experience struggle from time to time. We can see how the world views us versus how we see the world. We can give ourselves an intentional moment to create how we want to be in the world and how we want to resolve these conflicting messages.

As children age, they will likely hit another crisis as preteens or teens. In middle school or high school, children are conscious of body image and enter layers of dating and attractiveness. There can be a lot of pressure among teens to live up to an expected ideal and to feel wanted by and attractive to others. They may be also exploring their own sexuality, sexual identity, and sexual preferences. Having a hand that's different or wearing a prosthesis is different from the expected image. Sometimes this difference is welcomed and other times it is not. It is beneficial to intentionally teach your child effective coping strategies and work to build their self-esteem so they can feel confident navigating these messages and situations.

In the later teen and young adult years, children with limb differences tend to have more success resolving their identities and working on effective coping skills. As they continually build self-esteem and identity, healthy coping mechanisms developed in early childhood can extend into adulthood, supporting their ability to find pride in their body differences.

DISCUSSION QUESTIONS

Reflect on when your child first noticed their hand difference.

What was this experience like for them and for you?

Did you feel ready for your response?

What did you do?

What did you say?

If your child has not mentioned anything yet, what are ways you can respond?

IDENTITY DEVELOPMENT

Often, children with limb differences exist at an intersection of being able-bodied and disabled. Limb-different children tend to adapt to their body and their environment fairly well, becoming quite functional, which makes them viewed as more able-bodied in some situations. This can create a conflict where people with limb differences may feel that they do not belong in either the disability community or with the able-bodied community. Children with limb differences may claim to be a part of the disability community, only to find that others may retaliate, indicating that they are not truly disabled. Others may want to be part of the community but may not feel that they are "disabled enough." It is complicated, which makes all of the messaging difficult to figure out.

Many people haven't been exposed to someone with a hand difference and may not be educated about it. They only know that a child looks different. They don't have the same number of fingers or the same shape or size of arm. Their hands are questioned, often immediately pointed out and addressed. People automatically assume that children with differences can't do 2-handed tasks. How could they possibly ride a bike, or put up their hair, or work as a flight attendant? Society forgets that people are exceptionally adaptable.

The assumption that people with limb differences are unable to do everyday tasks means that larger society often views them under the broader scope of "disabled." In their view, disability is a bad thing, and these individuals are limited. However, there is more than one way to accomplish 2-handed tasks. Children and adults with hand differences are highly adaptable and find they can do the things they need to do and want to do. The way they do them may just look a bit different than expected. This is true with many members of the disability community; things will look different than expected, and this is OK!

If your parenting approach has been to identify the child as equally or exceptionally able, it's important to recognize that not everyone in society will foster the same view and that these messages can create conflict. In some ways, society will expect your child to fail and be surprised when they succeed. This leads to the overly inspiring messaging of people with differences and disabilities. This becomes problematic when society expects inspiration from people with disabilities. This has been called "inspiration porn"—a phrase coined by Stella Young, a disability activist. "Inspiration porn" describes the objectification of disabled people for the purposes of inspiring others. The underlying message says, "No matter how bad my life is, it could be worse. I could be disabled," which upholds the negative stigma on disability. The child may feel pressure to perform for others, to either prove or disprove societal expectations.

Recently, there has been work done by disability leaders and activists to generate pride around the terms "disability" and "disabled." Disability was the designation chosen by disabled leaders in the late 1980s and early 1990s, but there is a stigma associated with it. People have tried to get around the stigma by creating terms such as "differently-abled" or "specially-abled" or "uniquely-abled" or "differ-bility." These terms, however, uphold the stigma on disability. Be aware and mindful of when and how these terms are used. Who is using them? Are they terms used by people in the community? Or are they terms used by people who do not identify as a part of the community? Follow the language and insights spoken from those within the community.

Children without disabilities will uphold the messaging that disabilities are unfavored, and children with disabilities will feel this shift in messaging and realize that they have an unfavored trait. They may pick up on these microaggressions and acts of ableism and then believe them about themselves, which is called internalized ableism. Internalized ableism, or the idea that they cannot fully participate in society, may threaten a child's self-esteem and identity. This internalized thinking may limit what a child imagines they can or cannot do without even trying. If you're watching for this sort of behavior, listen to how they speak. For example, a child might say, "I don't have 2 hands. I can't climb the rock wall, swing on the monkey bars, or play that instrument." As a parent, explore pointing out the incorrect messaging with reflective questions such as, "What about the rock wall makes you think you can't climb it?" When the child responds with, "Because I don't have 2 hands," you can be ready to find alternative strategies to support them if they want to do this task. A child may engage in internalized ableism and limit their own ability to try out new things because they do not believe they can do the activity; they will not even try.

Your child may also hear positive or neutral messages about their hand difference from society at large. These messages may show up in social media or television or movies. Positive and negative messages make for truly inconsistent messaging. With so much conflicting information, children may become confused or develop social anxiety. They don't know how others will respond to them, and they become unsure how to handle it.

Children may feel the tension through messaging from parents and friends. Families may be saying, "You are normal; nothing is wrong with you," while society is telling them, "You are not normal; you can't do what we do." Children may struggle with their identity and the understanding of where they fit.

There are 2 narratives of disability. One is created by members of society who do not identify as disabled and have the perception that people with disabilities are "limited and unable." The second narrative comes from members of the disability community where they work to create the true and authentic experience of what it means to have a disability.

Disability is not a bad thing or a bad word, and people with disabilities can do the things they need to do and want to do, though they may need additional support or adaptations. They are just as important as any other members of society. Children with hand differences can grow into their disability identity, where they often find that their experiences are like others who have body differences. They can recognize that their hands are different from their peers; however, this difference is neutral. Their hand differences can be accepted as a piece of who they are. Children can be proud of their bodies and accept their adaptations.

Today, many groups are working to challenge perceptions on disability and to incorporate all disabilities into mainstream social norms. A significant amount of work remains to be done, but advocates make strides every day to help all children feel at home in a more inclusive social climate.

As children age, they will explore multiple identities, initially ones established by their parents and then gradually they will develop their own. Be conscious of similarities and differences in how you and your child identify with their abilities as they age. It is important to provide support and encouragement for your child as they grow up and be mindful of pressures and expectations. In the age of social media, some parents feel pressure to make their child "a limb-different superstar." Your child is already a superstar, so consider allowing them to choose if they want to be involved in the spotlight. Ensure that your child is the one controlling the narrative. They get to choose the words they want to describe themselves and how they want to tell their story. You, as a parent, can work together to help develop ideas but ultimately ensure their story comes from their perspective. Your story comes from your perspective, and you should feel like you can share your story if you wish. But be mindful of what is your story as a parent versus your child's story.

DISCUSSION QUESTIONS

Reflect on your own identity.

What components are important to you?

How are they different from your parents' perception of your identity?

Think about your child as they age. They will have similar building blocks to you but will also build their own. How can you best support them as they explore their own identity?

DEVELOPING AND SUPPORTING NATURAL TALENTS

Children will be motivated and inspired and want to do different things, and not do other things, from arts to sciences to sports to drama. There are multiple clubs, activities, and skills that your child will be interested in developing. It is important to recognize your child's natural talents and support their interests, just as any parent would for any child. If your child is very interested in dancing, water polo, horseback riding, piano, or art—encourage them. People with limb differences have done all these things successfully in their lives. They may need extra tools, adaptations, or extra practice to effectively engage in an activity, but success encouraged from a natural ability can build confidence and self-identity.

Be mindful of discouraging your child from certain activities solely on the assumption that they won't be able to participate due to their limb difference. That should not be the limitation. Support does exist to help your child figure out a way to do the activity. This is where you can check in with your school resources or your medical team, including surgeons, occupational therapists, and prosthetists. Maybe a surgical intervention can create a more effective grip, or a prosthetic can help support holding a tennis racquet, or adapted reins can be made to support horseback riding.

Know that your child will fail at tasks and know that failing is a part of learning new skills. Failing provides opportunities to challenge barriers and find creative ways to readapt. Your child is not confined to only playing soccer because they can't hold a tennis racket. Many children with congenital hand differences have gone on to play elite tennis, engage in competitive rock climbing, and play professional baseball and football. There are so many amazing possibilities! There are people who have limb differences who are professionals in various talent realms: actors, models, dancers, musicians, motivational speakers, weightlifters, lawyers, commercial artists, chefs, scientists, therapists, doctors, flight attendants, and Miss America pageant winners! They are all there because they want to be and are engaged in the activities they found interesting and were supported along the way.

CHAPTER SUMMARY

In this chapter, we learned:

- How a child's identity develops and unique aspects for children with limb differences
- About the models of disability and how they can inform how the world sees your child

Chapter 10

A Support System: Cultivating Relationships with Friends and Family

In this Chapter

IN THIS CHAPTER, WE WILL LEARN:

- How family systems play a role with your children
- How current siblings play a role in the identity and health of each other
- How to explore and consistently communicate to establish functional support systems

Thinking on the individual experiences of limb differences, society, and stigmas, we are looking to expand on these ideas and see how individual experiences impact family dynamics and experiences. Having a family is fun and beautiful and complex. Each family member is connected to, is dependent on, provides for, and has specific roles and relationships to all the other family members. Having limb differences will impact the family dynamics. Let's explore family systems theories to understand how limb differences do not exist in isolation.

FAMILY SYSTEMS THEORIES

Family can be an important source of structure for a child with a hand difference. At the same time, all family members will feel the impact of the limb difference.

Other siblings may be asking questions about their sibling with a limb difference; all family members may also feel the stares even when others are not staring at them.

Dr Murray Bowen was a psychiatrist who developed the family systems theory from his research and observations of family interactions. The family systems theory highlights the interaction and interdependence of family members. According to Bowen, the experience of difference/disability is not only the experience of the child with the hand difference but rather that of the entire family. Sustaining open communication among all family members with your child is important.

Some families have children with other types of differences and disabilities, such as autism, or Down syndrome, or cerebral palsy. All of these are elements and features of the family unit. The family will work through balancing needs and wants and addressing components of the differences and disabilities as needed.

DISCUSSION QUESTIONS

If you have more than 1 child, how have the siblings interacted so far?

What has surprised you about their relationship(s)?

What has been a beautiful moment for them?

YOUR CHILD'S SIBLINGS

According to Bowen's family systems theory, all members of the family will operate as part of the same emotional unit. Family members will feel, behave, and use similar thinking when interacting with the external environment. Children without congenital hand differences will experience how the other family members respond emotionally and model that behavior to those outside the family unit. Family members can model acceptance and use of appropriate language. As parents, you set the tone, and siblings will learn through your coping mechanisms. Siblings may have questions or not understand why the new baby's hand does not look like theirs; younger siblings may not understand why their older sibling has a hand difference. Take the time to answer their questions, remembering they may ask the same question multiple times as they are developing their own understanding. This helps them build a response for when others ask about their sibling's hands. Taking the time to practice can help them feel equipped to navigate conversations.

Siblings will be a part of the decision process for how you want your family to approach communicating the congenital hand difference. They will mirror the words you use to describe your child's hand and will have similar responses to yours when others ask. Often siblings will be advocates for children with congenital hand differences. They can help convey to new peers what their sibling can do. Siblings can help create a safe and welcoming space outside the family for a child with a hand difference. Have them practice social scripts with their sibling who has a hand difference or practice with you. If the difference is treated as "cool" by a sibling, friends and other children are more likely to follow suit. Siblings may also answer questions about the hand difference, and they'll likely respond with words they've heard their parents say. New people may ask a brother or sister, "What happened?" instead of asking the child with the limb difference. Everyone in the family should use the agreed-upon language and learn how to politely decline to discuss the hand difference.

DISCUSSION QUESTIONS

What have family dynamics been so far?

How have sibling dynamics been so far?

What behaviors, comments, or questions do you see from your other children?

What examples have you set that work well for your family?

Describe a family event that went well. What about it went well?

Describe a family event that did not go well. What about it did not go well?

How can you help make this better if this type of event arises again?

When everyone is busy, siblings are sometimes the ones who take on triage roles, helping take care of other siblings. Older siblings tend to take on more responsibilities and may assist parents with household or caregiver tasks such as preparing meals for younger kids or babysitting. They may even take on an added sense of responsibility or protectiveness for the sibling with a hand difference. Let siblings organically explore the roles they want to take; however, be open for conversations and ways for them to discuss their experiences in these roles and determine whether these are the responsibilities they want to assume.

Sometimes children with congenital hand differences receive more attention due to their condition, which can, in turn, create tensions with the other siblings. Do other children feel jealous or overlooked? Create time and space in your family to address needs, wants, and desires of all your children. Your child's congenital hand difference is a part of your family dynamics, but it is not the only part of your family, nor does it define it. Your family is bigger than one child's hand difference, and you may need to step back to ensure that you balance the needs of all family members.

DISCUSSION QUESTIONS

What have siblings experienced in relation to the hand difference?

What are ways that you as a parent can build in time and energy to be given to your other children? Think of 3 activities.

TWINS

The same family systems theory applies when discussing sibling relationships in twins. Twins or multiples require more support and resources in general. If 1 or both of the children have hand differences, you may feel like you're spending your life driving to doctors, sitting in waiting rooms, and covering costs of surgery. Family dynamics with twins may result in even more powerful relationships than other types of siblings. From the first moment of life, your child will have an immediate peer for mirroring, comparing, and celebrating, as well as a companion in social settings. Preparing and setting up systems that will be supportive and functional for you and your family will be essential.

WHEN FAMILIES ARE NEW PEOPLE: ADOPTION

What happens when you adopt a child with a hand difference? On top of having a hand difference, everything for your newest family member may be new. Your child may also be learning a new language or attending a new school. As you grow together, you will get a chance to show your new child what family and community is for you and how you support and love them. Advocating for them around their hand difference will naturally become part of that love and support.

EXTENDED FAMILY

Family members play another important role when it comes to support. Parents may rely on extended family members to help make decisions about medical care. Research has shown that when parents have support from extended family, they are better able to support their children. This might include help from family members with physical needs, such as childcare or meal preparation, or others who provide emotional support and advice. Whether it's that cousin who has always listened to your fears or your parent who has always offered wise counsel, be mindful that your family members may need to process the limb difference as well, on their own terms. If you find a trusted family member is a little hesitant, offer an opportunity to share why. You may never know what they are feeling for you and your child unless you ask.

Research has shown that at times grandparents may feel guilty that they did something wrong leading to their child having a baby with a limb difference. They may feel blame or anger toward the parent who is not their child. Or in some cases, they may not agree with your decisions with regard to care. Ensure open communication and discussions based on medical facts. Research by Dr Eileen Bradbury, a prominent research psychologist in children with physical differences, showed that kids who had the support of involved grandparents tended to do better. Grandparents provide stability for the entire family if they are involved.

DISCUSSION QUESTIONS

Who have been your most helpful family members?

Have there been any who surprised you with their reaction to your child's difference? Were any confused or upset?

Who has stepped up, supported you, or helped with childcare or a meal?

Who didn't react the way you expected? Are they open to communication?

If you find these relationships still valuable, how can you open or nurture communication?

NEW FRIENDS AND OLD FRIENDS

Friendships provide community, support, and connection and are inherently important in our lives. As a parent, you may have multiple sets or communities of friends. Some of your friends may have children already, or maybe you are friendly with others expecting new babies at similar times. It may be easy to share your child's hand difference with them, or it may feel strange. Be mindful of how these relationships have changed, if at all, when they learned of your child's hand difference. Do you find their comments supportive or limiting? You will have to assess the power you assign to the other person's opinions through your friendship and the trust you have in each relationship.

Parents may have had friends who were all pregnant together. Maybe you exercised together or attended the same prenatal classes. As each friend has their baby, they are reaching out to you and excitedly telling you about how perfect their child is. However, when having a child with a limb difference, you may feel guilt, shame, or jealousy as other parents have these seemingly "perfect" children. These feelings are normal. Know that every child is perfect, and every child is imperfect. Share as much or as little as you feel right in the moment.

DISCUSSION QUESTIONS

How do you respond to new and old friends when they express emotions with you?

What feels different?

What feels the same?

How does stigma contribute?

DEVELOPING FRIENDSHIPS

Just like their parents, children will have friends, too. Creating friendships is an important part of human development. Friendships at every stage of our lives help provide positive enrichment, companionship, and support to our lives. Whether your child has a limb difference or not, they will need to learn how to navigate meeting someone new. There will likely be a process of *being discovered*, making an *explanation*, and *acceptance* of their hand differences from their peers.

When children make new friends, it's typically important that they feel accepted. And it's also quite common that once a child has formed a peer relationship, those same friends become allies. Sometimes, friends forget that the limb difference exists, and when someone points it out, they respond with, "Oh, I don't think anything of it. That's just my friend." Friends become accustomed to adaptations and different ways their friends interact with the world, and it becomes a part of their new norm.

If we look at the 3 stages of meeting someone new for a child with a hand difference, we can start with the moment of discovery of the hand difference. Kids are curious and notice differences, sometimes politely, and sometimes in ways that can be hurtful or insensitive. Depending on your own child's natural personality, this discovery phase can fall along the spectrum of a relatively harmless experience or lead to increased social anxiety.

Children may want to hide their limb in pockets, behind their back, or under tables to delay this discovery aspect longer and attempt to pass as normal. This sort of behavior is a coping mechanism that children may use depending on the amount of emotional energy they have to navigate social interactions. Some children may really love to talk about their limb differences and find the conversations enjoyable. Others may not enjoy them as much and would rather avoid them. Some people may even have their friends or family explain for them. All are ways of coping with this interaction.

Your child may or may not develop social anxiety when meeting new people, just as any child may feel anxious meeting new people. They might have one negative experience that may lead to increased social anxiety. If they continue to experience difficulty in this area, these negative experiences can create barriers to friendships. Be mindful of your child's friendships. If your child can regularly name a few friends or a best friend they are likely OK.

An even more accurate question can be to ask who is "the meanest in the class." If your child readily names meanies, then it is worth exploring whether there is bullying going on at school. Teachers, administration, health care providers, and counselors can help assess and address any anxieties or fears in developing friendships. They may be able to monitor for bullying while providing tools and strategies for securing social connections with others. Through their experiences with kids with similar differences, they will be able to guide you and your child in navigating social interactions.

DISCUSSION QUESTIONS

Reflect on the interactions your child has with new children.

What does this look like?

How does your child behave?

How do the other children behave?

What are you proud of?

As children grow, you'll be able to help them better navigate typical situations with friends like minor disagreements or hurt feelings that may have nothing to do with their limb differences. Teaching strong skills now will give them confidence and a great foundation for the future.

There are many models of parenting, and most people unconsciously take a bit from each of these models. When a child is struggling with peer interactions, questions remain: How much should a parent intervene and protect their child? How much should they let the child experience on their own so they can become more aware and adapt to their social surroundings? We all know what overprotective parents look like, or even neglectful ones. Beyond those extremes, it's a continuous learning curve for most parents. Not all interactions will be perfect, and you will learn from many of them. Remaining aware of your behavior and its impact on the child is a great place to start.

DATING AND RELATIONSHIPS

You may wonder what your child's road beyond elementary school might look like. The good news is that it looks much like any other teenager or college student or new young adult's journey. As parents, you want to protect your child, and those emotions won't change when they begin to date or have relationships.

People with limb differences are in all types of relationships. You can feel secure knowing that if your child wants to be in a relationship, your child will. They may establish relationships with someone who has similar—or dissimilar—physical differences. Or they may meet someone with no physical differences at all. A child with limb differences may travel through all different types of relationships over time. Some limb-different adults have dated several people, some have been married for a long time, and many are parents and great-grandparents. All of them have navigated the skills needed to go out on a first date, begin and end relationships, meet in-laws, parent children, feed babies, push strollers, support their families financially, and surround themselves with love, all while having a limb difference.

The right people will want to hold your child's hand and respect that it is a part of them, not something to be looked down upon or feel uneasy about. Adults with limb differences may have hands that are less accessible to wedding rings and come up with creative solutions. They wear their rings on the opposite hand, wear them on necklace chains, wear anklets, or skip rings all together. Some couples find other symbols of commitment to their partner. There are a variety of possibilities, and your child and their partner will choose what is best for them.

Some teens and adults with limb differences have anecdotally shared that sometimes people are "weird" about the hand difference, make a big deal about it, or do not want to date the person with a limb difference. However, most adults with hand differences also appreciate that their hand difference helps identify very quickly people who they do not want in their lives—like a social superpower.

Depending on the child's experience or barriers encountered when building friendships, they may have decreased self-esteem and increased insecurities. Help to remind your child that they are worthy of dating people who will love them and support them, that they do not have to date the first person who gives them attention. Help your child determine if the attention feels genuine and work with them to decide if they are even interested in dating that person. Teens may also be exploring their sexual preferences, sexual expressions, and multiple roles and identities. This may make dating a little more complicated. Work to support your child's self-esteem and confidence and help your child develop the skills to seek out partners who are beneficial for them.

CHAPTER SUMMARY

In this chapter, we learned:

- About the science and family dynamics of siblings
- That you can feel empowered to model behaviors you want others to have with your child
- That you can share as much or as little as you like with family and community
- That you are not responsible for anyone's feelings and can end conversations at any time

Chapter 11

Branching Out: Finding Community

In this Chapter

IN THIS CHAPTER, WE WILL LEARN:

- About various types of communities that exist for parents of and children with hand differences
- About support that can be found in communities
- How to determine what types of communities are right for you and your family

As you continue to explore parenting a child with a hand difference, you'll find that your child's needs—and yours—extend beyond the medical world and the friendships you have developed so far. As you embark on this journey, you will find there is value in the communities you find along the way.

Communities connect us and help us feel seen and understood by others. They allow us to learn from others who share something similar. Communities shape who we are, from neighborhoods and schools, to sports and hobbies, to religion and music. Communities help us interconnect and relate to others with similar experiences. They help us feel less alone.

We as humans live complex lives and find our needs may be best met as members of many communities. Having a child with a limb difference is rare enough that you may find yourselves to be the only parents you know in a similar situation. You may have a supportive family or care team but still feel that no one "gets" you. Please know that other families are feeling this, too!

The good news is that there are other parents, children, teens, and adults with hand differences who may be beneficial as you develop a supportive community of your own. Whether they are new parents or have grown children, you may want to meet them, hear their stories, and discuss each of your celebrations, worries, and decisions.

Whether you create your own community or find a group ready for you, having contact with other parents can help reassure you that you and your family will be just fine. You might even pick up some advice on how to teach your child 1-handed shoe tying or talk with your partner or co-parent. You may find yourself providing advice, support, and comfort to other parents who have children with limb differences.

As you grow with your communities, you'll find that they become forums for you to celebrate milestones and find comfort when you might not feel like the most perfect of parents. Each support system has something to give you, and you have something to give to each one.

Fortunately, with the advent of the internet and social media, communities are more accessible than ever. Multiple types of limb-different communities exist across many areas of the internet, which means you can find the ones that work best should you or your family want to be a part of them.

Depending on your location and proximity to in-person services, you may also have a wider variety of available options. Larger cities or those with major children's hospitals will, by their nature, offer more services in addition to social media and online forums via limb-different organizations. Communities can generally fall into a few broad categories:

- Those for parents and close family members
- Those providing resources and advocacy on behalf of those with limb differences
- Those for the kids themselves

Within each broad category, groups can be found in a variety of places:

- Medical and patient communities
- Group therapy
- Social media groups and online forums
- Resource and advocacy organizations
- Camps
- Events
- Self-organized get-togethers

As you explore the world of communities, there is a rule to keep in mind. Your community should make you feel empowered. Sometimes, members of these groups can seem opinionated or even unsupportive. Group dynamics don't always bring out the best in people, and some parents express themselves in a way you may find hurtful. Recognize that every parent processes emotions differently, but also take care of your own feelings. If you don't feel that you're getting the support and community from a group, consider finding a new community that will better fit your style and your needs.

Think of a community as a give and take—you gain knowledge and insight and give your own support and care. But when the balance starts to tip too far in one direction or the other, you might want to examine if it's still a healthy experience for you. Communities are not exact in their natures—and they grow and evolve. If they do not make you or your child feel more confident, perhaps reconsider participating.

DISCUSSION QUESTIONS

Reflect on the first community you found, and describe how you felt the first time you told a supportive community about your child's congenital hand difference.

What new questions did this community create or answer?

What support did you feel?

What do you want from a community?

What can you contribute to a community?

MEDICAL AND PATIENT COMMUNITIES

Most clinicians recognize that finding support for the patient or their family is just as important as medical treatment. And most patients—and parents of patients—would say that they have many more questions than sometimes their doctors or care teams can answer. For these reasons, many hospitals and even doctors can recommend on-site groups to you. You may want to hear about experiences from other nearby families who are living similar milestones right in your neighborhood. When you hear parents talk about kids of different ages who have hand differences, you may recognize the need for sharing your story. Check with your doctor or other care professionals to see if you can be informed of local, in-person support services, perhaps with hospital sponsorship.

GROUP THERAPY

Group therapy is one way that parents—or children—can safely share their experiences and feelings with others who may feel the same or have experienced similar situations. Moderated by a professional, some groups can be condition specific, while others may include children with a variety of differences. Some groups may even be specifically for parents of children going through certain major surgeries or long hospital stays.

Moderators in group therapy settings are therapists trained in guiding and responding to topics discussed. These groups typically meet regularly and have clearly defined goals. The facilitator will provide resources and tools to support and guide individuals in their journey. These groups are spaces to help support parents as much as needed and are typically run in hospitals or universities. Groups can be found by internet search or asking your health care team for recommendations or referrals to group therapy.

DISCUSSION QUESTIONS

What support would you want from others who are in a similar place?

What information or connection do you think would be beneficial for you or your child, if any?

SOCIAL MEDIA GROUPS

Social media platforms are useful ways for people with common interests to connect. Whether they're broad public communities or more private "gated communities" like pages, invitation-only groups, chatrooms, or photo or video communities, they can provide virtual spaces to ask questions and learn from other parents of children with hand or limb differences.

Groups on these platforms can be specific to a condition like Poland syndrome or can be specific to a region like "West Coast congenital limb-different group." This helps to provide a live connection to other parents of children and adults living with hand differences. Be sure to review the group's mission, culture, and rules for posts and responses. And know that sometimes people can be very opinionated. There is more than one way to raise a child. There may be learning moments communicating with those different perspectives. Engage with the communities that provide you the most support!

You can generally find these groups by searching on any given platform for hashtags or terms such as "limb difference," "limb difference awareness," "hand difference," or "no arms," or by a specific diagnosis such as "symbrachydactyly," "amniotic band syndrome," or "cleft hand."

You can also use social media platforms to follow parents of and adults living with hand differences as they navigate the world. Their profiles often show their daily activities and adaptations they've made as well as their thoughts and feelings. Keep in mind that the accounts may be personal and/or professional, and content and content appropriateness will vary. Some may even advocate a specific treatment, technique, or affiliation with a group. You may want to review the accounts and look for the messages that both seem to differ and align with your family's perspective and values.

Be mindful that everyone is on their own journey with their hand difference experience and that they may have different messaging. Always feel free to "follow" or "unfollow" or "re-follow" accounts at any time. You can read messages, watch their videos, and engage with what they are sharing, but ultimately you are the one who gets to decide what messages are valuable to you and your family.

DISCUSSION QUESTIONS

What are positive messages you have received from social media accounts?

What are negative messages you have received?

What are things you have learned from social media accounts?

What do you want from social media accounts?

Are there any accounts that are not helpful for you or your family that you may want to reconsider following?

RESOURCE AND ADVOCACY ORGANIZATIONS

There are several organizations, both for-profit and not-for-profit, that exist to provide resources as well as a voice for different communities both locally and globally. Some are specific to upper limbs, while others are broader and cover differences to both upper and lower limbs, whether acquired or congenital. These organizations will be clear about their mission and vision, showing the direct use of donated funds on their website and in their materials. If they're not, exercise caution.

Some organizations raise funds for research or patient support, some provide information on surgeries and prosthetics, and others may offer scholarships or grants to help cover costs. Still, others provide legislative information and actively lobby the government, while others hold community gathering events or create merchandise for limb-different pride. Some organizations provide constant connection and offer families and advocates a variety of support groups and online forums, while others don't. And frankly, some groups have goals which you may or may not agree with. When joining or supporting an organization, make sure you determine which ones align with your family's point of view and need for support. These organizations can be found by using internet search words of "amputee organizations" and "limb difference organizations." Some organizations will have a resources page that will list other organizations; you can search around and find the organizations that meet your and your family's needs. These organizations likely have social media accounts affiliated with them, and you can consider following them if they meet your needs and you like to be connected on social media platforms.

CAMPS

Camps can be a great activity for kids (and even the entire family if it's a family camp) that provides a safe, supportive environment for children with limb differences. These camps can be day or sleepaway camps, usually in the summer, and they're often sponsored by hospitals or organizations to try to connect children in similar situations. Camps can be narrowly focused to congenital upper limb patients of the host hospital. Camps can also be for children with broad-based limb differences, where campers can have upper/lower, congenital, and acquired limb differences. Camps can also be open to children with various kinds of disabilities. Children get a chance to socialize in a safe environment and meet kids with similar differences. It gives kids a chance to try new things.

Summer camps can have specific themes such as sports camps or therapy camps. Some are for-profit where families pay a fee, while others are hosted through not-for-profit organizations, making them free for families. Some organizations offer scholarships to sponsor travel and camp costs.

To find camps, search online for "limb difference summer camps" or ask your hospital, support group, or friends who have children with limb differences. Most camps tend to host children from 7 to 17 years old, although some may take younger children for a shorter duration. You might also research "family camps" for the entire family to see if any work for you.

EVENTS

As you research your support and community options, you'll also find a wide variety of events that have been organized by other parents. They may be called "outings" or "weekends." Some are for the entire family, and others for parents or children alone. Picnic days are afternoon events for the whole family. Children can play games and mingle while parents can connect with other parents. Get-togethers often offer lots of good mentor opportunities and various exposures to new tools, devices, resources, merchandise, or connections. These picnic days can be organized by professional organizations or parents themselves.

Check testimonials to see if the organization fits your family's needs. Feel free to connect with parents who attend prior to the event beginning. This may help you to feel somewhat prepared before registering. Travel and financial support may be needed to attend these events depending on location. Some organizations offer financial support, or families can sponsor each other.

You may also find professionally organized events created by organizations that have the goals of education, resources, and advocacy. These might include guest speakers or lecture series, informal coffees, online video meetups, or even evening events that are fun nights out. These types of organizations typically involve professionals who are knowledgeable about the topics discussed. They can include events hosted by your child's hospital and may include guest speakers and resources for development. Other organizations may host highly organized sports for children with differences and may give awards or medals to top competitors.

If you are involved with any organizations, associations, or advocacy groups, you may also find that you are often invited to fundraisers. Some are family oriented, while others provide parents an opportunity for some time on their own. If you feel strongly about the mission or value of an organization, supporting it financially may be something that interests you. If you're not able to make (or interested in making) a large gift, that is OK. You can support the group via a fundraising event that gives you the opportunity to meet parents and families with similar experiences. And many of these groups raise money to help make research and advocacy possible. As with all groups, do your research and follow your instincts. Whether it's a walk-a-thon or a carnival, these kinds of fundraisers and events can be fun ways for your entire family to participate together and show their support.

DISCUSSION QUESTIONS

If you could meet a group of parents whose children with hand differences are grown up, what would you ask them?

What questions would you have for the adult with hand differences?

SELF-ORGANIZED GET-TOGETHERS

Self-organized get-togethers may have a lot of similarities in structure and benefit to their professionally organized counterparts. These events are created by parents who want to build a space for families to meet each other. Maybe it's a small picnic with a few families or a few vendors. Since these sorts of events are self-organized, they can make parents feel empowered to host them for their own communities.

Ultimately, remember that you are building your own community, and you can choose the people you gather around you. Every person, every child, and every family is unique, and everyone is at a different stage of their own journey. As you listen to what people say, remember that you have the power to integrate their advice or not. Be mindful of what messages are being shared and how they align with your messaging. What can be learned from all these messages?

People you encounter in support and advocacy groups may have strong opinions, and oftentimes they can be polarizing. You yourself may have strong opinions that differ from the group. Remember that there is very rarely one way to do something, and very rarely do people have to do something a certain way.

You are the expert of yourself. Your family is the expert of your family. Your child is the expert of their experience. Look for the spaces where you can find support and the spaces where you can learn from others' experiences. If you find that messaging is not helpful, feel empowered to unsubscribe from it. Know that being a member of these groups is fluid—you may attend 1 event a year, or you may find that you've outgrown a group or the group has evolved in a different way. You and your family may want support from one type of group at one time and then may need support from another type of group at another time. These communities exist and will always exist for whatever duration you need them. Feel free to float in and out of them over the years, and feel empowered to create your own to fill the needs you have. It is all about what works best for you and your family.

CHAPTER SUMMARY

In this chapter, we learned:

- How to explore various types of communities that can help support you and your child
- The benefits of each type of group
- That you can be a part of lots of different types of groups
- How different groups will have different messaging and to be mindful of the context of messages
- That group membership can be fluid, and you can flow between the groups as much as you and your family needs

Chapter 12

Adapting Advocacy: Navigating School and the Government

In this Chapter

IN THIS CHAPTER, WE WILL LEARN:

- Things to consider when starting school
- What resources you can and should expect from teachers and school systems
- Policies that support employment and where to access them

Now that we have discussed friendships and communities, let's talk about government policies and how they are developed to support your child in the things they need and want to do. In this section, we will cover resources and strategies to help you and your child feel more prepared to dive into the world of new friends, arts and crafts, and games at recess until they get their first jobs and become adults in the world. Policies have been written to ensure they are supported and free of discrimination along the way.

ENTERING SCHOOL

Parents and children with or without limb differences have a lot of excitement, and sometimes some separation anxieties, when it comes to starting school for the first time. Give space to develop a good platform of confidence and communication skills. It will be easier for your child to field the "What happened to your hand?" question as they meet new people. These introductions can feel uncomfortable since we are all unsure of how new people will respond. Knowing that you and your family are in control of the words you want to use when talking about your child and their hand difference can help. For a review, draw from the social scripts in Chapter 4, and role play with your child if they feel anxious about meeting a whole new set of peers.

Teachers may not be familiar with the needs of children with congenital limb differences and may look to the parent for advice on how to best support the child. Teachers are often open to meetings prior to the start of school to address any concerns. These meetings can be beneficial, as your child can show off their adaptive strategies and familiarize the teacher with these skills. When your teacher is supportive of the adaptive strategy of your child, say using their elbow to hold a cup, for example, it normalizes the adaptation for others as well.

CONSIDERATIONS OF PROSTHESIS USE

It is recommended for the child to begin school, or any new environment, interacting with objects as they did prior to the first day of school. This will set the child up to feel empowered to participate joyfully. If your child uses prosthetic devices at home, bring them to school if they are helpful. However, it is not recommended for a child to start using a prosthesis and enter a new school environment at the same time. Work to try to stage both of these brand-new activities.

If your child uses prostheses, intermittently check in with the teacher on the role of these prosthetic devices and adaptive equipment in the child's day, and help support them to make changes along the way as needed. Provide the teacher with instructions as to when devices should be put on or taken off and how devices should be taken on and off to maintain their function. Help the teacher develop guidelines and search for cues for when the device is being used beneficially as a tool and when the device is being used less beneficially and as a toy.

THE FIRST TEACHER MEETING

When you first meet with your child's new teacher, you may want to consider topics to be covered and information you'd like to ensure you share with them. Many of the strategies we've already discussed can help. You can outline the conversation you want to have with the teacher by starting with an information sheet. Here are some sample conversation points:

> **Medical background of the congenital hand difference**
> Share with your child's teacher any of the diagnostic criteria or background that you have learned about your child and their hand difference.

"My daughter was born with aphalangia, which means that her left hand ends in nubbins at her knuckles. We do not know why this happened, and it is not a result of anything we did or did not do."

The words your family uses for the hand difference

"We like to use the words 'limb difference' or 'leftie' when we talk about her hand; please use these words also and help teach her classmates that these are the terms used."

How your family introduces the congenital hand difference with other children

"When kids start asking about her hand, we say, 'That's part of who she is; she has brown hair, green eyes, and a hand difference. Sometimes hands look like this.'"

Show off/demonstrate

Show off or demonstrate different tasks, such as building with blocks, carrying items, opening containers, putting on shoes and jackets, and writing. This familiarizes your child's teacher with how your child has already made adaptations and modifications. Your child's teacher can then anticipate these differences and help educate your child's classmates as part of the classroom experience.

Different tasks that your child may need support with and how to help your child best

"My daughter is still working on zipping up her jacket. She may need help getting the zipper started; once it is started, she doesn't usually need additional help."

Things your child likes to do

"My daughter loves to dance, she takes ballet lessons, and she loves horses."

Your concerns, so that you can work with the teacher to develop a plan to address them

"I am concerned with how her peers will interact with her hand since school-aged kids notice her difference; she was teased recently on the playground. How do you manage teasing in the classroom?"

Features of adaptive equipment or prosthetic devices

Share with your child's teacher the purpose, features, and management of the equipment and devices as well as instructions you have told your child to do when using/caring for devices.

"My son uses a prosthesis for tasks when he is sitting at a desk for things like writing and cutting, but he tends to take it off when running outside. There might be some redness right when he first takes it off; however, the skin should not be broken, have sores, or be visibly

irritated, and the redness should fade away quickly. If these things happen, refrain from putting the prosthesis back on and please tell a nurse and have them call me."

"This is called a splint, and it fits between my daughter's thumb and her palm. It is to help widen this space. She is supposed to wear it at night, but she likes it and may bring it to school. It is hard plastic and will melt if left in the sun or on a heater. She knows she is not supposed to bring it to school because we don't want to lose it or break it. Please take it if you see it, and we can come to pick it up later."

Any additional information that is helpful for your child's teacher to know
Ask your child's teacher if they have any questions.

SCHOOL-BASED THERAPY

There are a number of federal policies established to support children with disabilities in the classroom. These services may or may not benefit your child. All schools that receive federal funding will provide school-based therapy. These therapy services are up to each state and even the school districts on how they are enforced or carried out. This means there is a wide variation from school to school, and some systems and districts may have access to more resources than others. Some schools may have therapists who are employed directly by the school, while others will hire contract therapists or will offer therapy services at a separate location. If you have befriended a family in another school, you might be concerned because things aren't the same in your school as theirs. Policies may differ from school to school, so talking with other parents in your same school district can be important in your school decisions. Lean on your team of supporters and allies (teachers, physicians, therapists, case managers, school counselors, family, and friends) to help you navigate tricky policies. Researching these resources will be something you may consider as you look at school options for your child.

ASSESSMENTS

Teachers screen and evaluate students to ensure they are meeting learning objectives and progressing throughout the year. If they find that a child might qualify for a standardized assessment, they will request one. A standardized assessment will identify any areas where targeted interventions may help. It is a research-based skills test with measures to determine if your child can perform certain tasks compared with other children of the same age. For example, an assessment might measure your child's independence when using the bathroom at school, writing, and cutting with scissors. Assessments may review developmentally appropriate gross motor skills, fine motor skills, comprehension, and independence.

When you have an initial meeting with your child's teachers, talk with them about your child's progress. If you as a parent feel that your child may benefit from further evaluation, or if you feel your child's needs are not being met, you have the right to request an assessment/evaluation from your school administration.

If an assessment determines that your child would benefit from interventions, they may be eligible to receive adaptations, modifications, and therapeutic services such as occupational therapy. These services are provided under 2 federal laws: Section 504 of the Rehabilitation Act of 1973 and the Individualized Educational Plan (IEP) from the Individuals with Disabilities Education Act (IDEA). Knowing what to ask for by name can assist in your advocacy efforts for your child if needed.

Section 504

A plan under Section 504 (often called a "504 plan" or simply a "504") deals specifically with accommodations and modifications for the physical needs your child might have. Section 504 is the policy that applies to the school setting to ensure that children with a documented disability and documented needs receive accommodations to access the learning environment and curriculum. If the student needed a slant board, a pencil grip, or a particular seating arrangement, those accommodations could be provided as part of the plan. Children with congenital limb differences will likely receive services covered by this policy.

You, your child, your child's teacher, and other school professionals will develop a collaborative team. This team will meet and develop a plan to implement modifications and accommodations that have been determined to support your child in school. The team will agree and is legally responsible to carry out the accommodations and modifications determined in the meeting. Your child will be monitored for progress to determine if the supports are no longer needed or if modifications to the plan are required. Schools are mandated to provide these services under 504 but are not federally reimbursed for the cost of accommodations or modifications made in compliance.

IEP

If your child needs an IEP, it will relate specifically to barriers to educational and learning progress and address supports to access the school curriculum. An IEP is mandated by IDEA, which is federal legislation separate from Section 504. The IEP is designed to support children's learning. For children to qualify for services, the child must have a documented disability that falls under a specific category covered by the legislation and have documented educational needs and learning difficulties.

Then, you, your child, your child's teacher, and other educational professionals involved meet to determine a detailed individualized plan with learning goals to support your child most effectively. This plan will be reviewed annually to determine if learning goals have been met, if new ones need to be created, or if services are no longer needed. Federal funds reimburse IEP services. Under an IEP plan, children may receive ongoing therapy services with goals that are developed and intended to be met within 1 year. If the child is not progressing or is progressing too quickly, any one of the team members is legally required to call a new IEP meeting to review goals and create ones that are appropriate. The child is required to be reevaluated every 2 years to determine qualifications for therapy.

GETTING HIRED AND STARTING CAREERS

People with limb differences are successfully employed in a wide variety of professions, working as servers, flight attendants, actors, professional weightlifters, motivational speakers, mechanics, scientists, artists, doctors, nurses, researchers, and lawyers. The concern, however, can include discrimination, which can be a reality. Know and ensure that your child knows that federal law prevents employers from asking specific interview questions about their limb difference. Employers are not allowed to discriminate against the hand difference if the person is able to complete all job functions with reasonable accommodations; this is covered under the Americans with Disabilities Act of 1990.

Let's break down that sentence a bit further. Every job post has a list of required duties. Your child will review these duties and identify if any of these may be potential barriers; you can review these with them if they want support. Reasonable accommodations include adaptations that an employer is required to make to help an individual gain access to a job, like more complete dictation software or an adaptive desk setup. You can find job accommodations and support via internet searches or talking with human resources. There are typing programs that exist if your child is interested in increasing speed, advanced software adaptations for voice-only services, or even 1-handed typing maps to assist with efficient keyboarding. Accommodations by the employer are federally required for their employees; however, they are not federally reimbursed for these accommodations.

The topic of disclosure—telling a potential employer about a disability—can be tricky, but legally, no one can make your child disclose a disability. Depending on the job, disclosing a hand difference means the employer can make accommodations for the job but may open the door to discrimination as well. Talk it out with your child and help support them in the decision that works best for them. If your child is experiencing discrimination in the workplace, they can file reports to their managers or human resources or take legal action by seeking out guidance and counsel from disability lawyers.

Teens and adults with hand differences have been successfully employed and work at all kinds of jobs in all kinds of industries. Encourage your child to explore and try out different jobs and careers just as you would any other child. If your child is feeling anxious about their ability to, say, carry a serving tray or manage gloves and fine motor medical equipment, find ways they can practice at home until they feel confident in their abilities and know what adaptations they may need. Your child may benefit from vocational rehabilitation that supports job training and job exploration and may have scholarships/funding available for a given career field. Connect with case managers or search for vocational rehabilitation centers in your community. Teens/adults with limb differences can always ask to practice things in the work environment as well; this is a reasonable accommodation.

Not every child is going to be amazing at every job, and there may be limitations and expectations on job functions that prevent any number of people from getting jobs. However, support your child's natural talents and interests. Work with them to figure out ways to attain that job or career or the closest thing they can to it. Encourage your child to follow their interests and talents; there is always a way.

BECOMING THEIR OWN ADVOCATE

As children grow into adulthood, they will likely go on to lead independent lives. Independence looks different from adult to adult, and some adults may need more support than others. As a child who may need extra support and adaptations is gearing up to live more independently, it is important to consider various topics and find ways to practice these supports while they are still at home.

Make sure they are aware of their own medical records and care. You may have already experienced this transition, as medical professionals are required to work directly with patients when they turn 18. (In fact, it may come as a surprise the first time the doctor tells you that they've shared information directly with your child that they didn't share with you.) As your child takes control of their own medical care, they may be transitioning to new health insurance providers available, for example, on college campuses or at employee health centers, registering for their own doctors, and transferring medical records. They need a list of current medications, family history of illnesses, allergic reactions, and documentations of therapeutic, surgical, or prosthetic interventions. Ensure they have complete understanding of information about their congenital hand difference. They may ask you about circumstances surrounding pregnancy, birth, and dates of surgeries, as well as types of prosthetic devices and any continuing care they may need. Often, early interventions that occurred when they were young are important. If you have kept your notes or your organizational system from their toddler years, you can share those with them. Share your thoughts and your decision making. Re-explain events so their adult selves can understand them and the context in which the interventions took place. They may be aware of a surgery they had at 8, but their 8-year-old understanding will be different than their 21-year-old understanding; re-explain it to them as adults.

Your child may need additional support and adaptations to live independently, depending on their needs. They may no longer have you to help turn on showers, prep ingredients for a recipe, or drive them places. If your child has a goal of moving out on their own, work toward proficiency in these activities of daily living. They should feel comfortable living on their own and know how to find assistance, support, or services when they need them. If applicable, you can request occupational therapy services to help your grown-up child address any types of independent living skills or set up living environments to help promote more independent living as needed.

Help your child create a support system if they need someone at any point. If they're moving to another city or region, help them identify relatives or trusted friends who can serve as points of contact. You can also help them find agencies and services that can assist with anything that might come up. Maybe their new apartment has stairs, and carrying up large items is difficult. Or perhaps managing light switches while carrying items in and out of apartments may be tricky. Once they know the barriers, they can look for alternative strategies, such as backpacks or carts that have wheels designed to climb up stairs or smart home systems with voice-activated controls for lights and music.

Your child may learn about becoming their own advocate by connecting with fellow limb-different humans and the disability community. When they live on their own for the first time, they may have limited support to help them navigate new relationships and new people. They may encounter microaggressions and internalized ableism that they've not encountered since they were younger. Combined with new experiences, a new job, a new university program, or even a new family, it may take some time to process these things and may feel exhilarating and sometimes overwhelming. While celebrating these milestones of young adulthood, help remind your child of effective coping, and establish support within their new environment that can assist them.

Remind your child that they can access or contact disability services (if at a school) or human resources (if working) to help establish connections, understand their experience, and provide support and services if necessary.

There are thousands of adults living independently with limb differences who have all their wants fulfilled and needs met. You and your grown-up child are going to be just fine.

CHAPTER SUMMARY

In this chapter, we learned:

- How to provide strategies for creating alliances with teachers and peers in the classroom
- How to understand school-based 504 and IEP therapy plans and how your child may qualify for services
- How to think about some of the additional unique steps for independence and self-care ahead in your child's young adulthood

Chapter 13

Creating Your Own Hand Book

In this *Hand Book*, we hope that you have found resources, sample discussion questions to ask yourself, and up-to-date information to consider. Take from it what you find helpful, leave the things that are not useful or that you are not interested in. Welcoming and raising children is an up-and-down and in-and-out journey. You may want to revisit sections of this book over time and review the information and concepts that are important or shifting at those future moments along the way.

We encourage you to use the blank pages at the end of this book to help outline and guide your process and progress. Chapter titles in *The Hand Book* can be your guide, along with each chapter's discussion questions. Write down what you found most helpful or important in creating your personalized, very own resource that is tailored to you and your family's individual needs. The references at the end of this book can be used for additional reading if you want to dive deeper into any of the topics covered throughout the chapters.

If you've read this far, then you are well on your way to becoming knowledgeable, resourced, and empowered parents of a child with a hand difference. We are on this journey with you!

Acknowledgments

This book would not exist without the children with hand differences and their families that we've both met over these years. We sincerely thank you. We have tremendous gratitude for everyone involved and know that this would not be possible without your support, mentorship, and critical and thoughtful review. You are the giants' shoulders that we stand on. We would like to thank those who provided countless hours of reading, editing, writing, long conversations on the nuances of topics, and lengthy discussions of word choice throughout this project. Thank you to the American Society for Surgery of the Hand (ASSH) and American Foundation for Surgery of the Hand (AFSH) for the opportunity to work alongside you and create accessible content for parents and patients. Thank you to Renee Wilmeth, Molly Aaron, and Kendall Steinle for your work in development editing. Thank you to Meredith Boe for your expert copyediting. Thank you to Lauren Wheeler for your thoughtful reorganizational work and bringing together the medical and empathetic voices. Thank you most to Olivia Williams for your amazing organization, valued contributions, and critical guidance as we navigated publication.

Nina Lightdale-Miric, MD
Sarah Tuberty, OTD, OTR/L

Thank you foremost to the patients and families who have allowed me the privilege of caring for and learning from them. I am so grateful to the generous CATCH supporters, including Vivian Feintech, Arleen S. Gamza, Jonny Savic, the Mirics, the Silvermans, the Smiths, the Helen and Jose Colton Foundation, 8 awesome CATCH-Princeton research interns, the Children's Hospital Los Angeles (CHLA) Foundation staff, and the many others who have sustained this meaningful, impactful program for its first decade. Thank you to my parents, Reina and Charles, and 3 sisters, Jenifer, Hallie, and Sarah—our family is the foundation of all that I value and build on every day. Thank you to Sharon Everson, my first coach, who taught me how to do the work to be my best self through all the wins and losses. I am tremendously indebted to my teachers and professors at Princeton University, Dartmouth Medical School, Duke Medicine, and the Hospital for Special Surgery. Most notably, thank you to Drs James R. Urbaniak, Milan Stevanovic, Marybeth Ezaki, Myles Cohen, Peter Waters, and Don Bae for their inspirational mentorships. Thank you Phyllis D'Ambra, RN for your vision. Thank you to my supportive department chairs, Vernon Tolo, David Skaggs, Robert Kay, and David Kulber, my inspiring pediatric orthopedic surgery partners, the talented Joan Wright, the formidable Allison Tarrasch, cool cat Monica Rizzo, the invaluable nurses Ann Wakulich, Cathy Salata, Elaine Butterworth, and Amelita Quiton, the wonderful occupational therapists, and most caring staff at CHLA for all their teamwork and dedication. Thank you, Sarah Tuberty, my true co-conspirator; this little idea of a book took years of intentional dedication and open communication. Finally, and full-heartedly, thank you to Alex, Peter, and Helena. You 3 are my reasons.

Nina Lightdale-Miric, MD

Thank you Dr Michelle James for caring for me and my family from day 1; thank you for answering all of our questions and for empowering my parents to raise me. Thank you for your continued mentorship and support. Thank you to Janice Conroy and Sally Martens for your big hearts and insightful guidance. When I struggle with navigating the world, you both remind me through your own examples that "you will never regret being kind." To Ginny Gibson for giving your free time to directing Camp Winning Hands and to Tal Oppenheimer and Tessa Artale as fierce planning committee partners. Ellen Cohn, Jessica Kramer, John Kramer, Jennifer Kalenburg, and Karen Jacobs for your mentorship, thoughtful questions, and support, and challenging me to think deeper in graduate school. Sabrina, Matt, Simoine, and Lydia Orlando for welcoming me into your family and supporting me to write this text. To Nicole Kelly, who is the most incredible cheerleader, thank you for helping me find my disability pride and for growing the fire in my belly to create positive change. To Danny Jordan for your powerful insight and for creating mindful and impactful resources for the community. To Kevin Herbert for your input and review. To my parents, Katheryn and Dennis, my sister, Madeline Tuberty, and my partner, Erik Brewer, for your laughs, love, and support and for encouraging me to chase my dreams all around the world.

Thank you, Nina, for having this idea, and for inviting me into the project in the summer of 2019. I am appreciative of our partnership and our thoughtful dialogue, and I am proud to work with you on this project.

Thank you to all of the families who have shared their stories with us; we listened to them and carried them with us as we wrote this text. Know that your stories are providing empathy and acceptance to new parents of children with hand differences every day.

Thank you to all of the brave and fierce children, teens, and adults living with limb differences.

We are proud of you and hope to do right by you.

Sarah Tuberty, OTD, OTR/L

About the Authors

NINA LIGHTDALE-MIRIC, MD, a graduate of Princeton University and Dartmouth Medical School, completed an orthopedic surgery residency at Duke University, followed by a fellowship in hand and upper extremity surgery at the Hospital for Special Surgery in New York with subspecialty pediatric and congenital hand surgery training at Boston Children's Hospital, Texas Scottish Rite Hospital for Children, Institut de la Main in Paris, and Ilizarov Center in Kurgan.

As a board-certified orthopedic pediatric hand surgeon at CHLA, Dr Lightdale-Miric sees approximately 100 patients and their families each week in her hospital clinic and performs more than 300 surgeries per year. She is an associate professor at the University of Southern California Keck School of Medicine, teaching undergraduate and graduate classes. She teaches and trains future generations of pediatric hand surgeons at CHLA and Cedars-Sinai Medical Center.

CATCH—the Center for Achievement of Teens and Children with Hand Differences—was initiated in 2010 after Dr Lightdale-Miric observed that the parents of her patients were exchanging information in the hallways and waiting rooms. Children with hand differences wanted to meet each other. She and Phyllis D'Ambra, RN, decided to see who would show up if they held a picnic to give families an opportunity to connect, with a goal of also presenting a relevant educational program. A perfect venue was available at CHLA, but an event would be costly. This problem was solved, as Dr Lightdale-Miric was about to be married. She and her husband, Dr Alexander Miric, decided to accept donations instead of wedding gifts, and all the proceeds went to a fund at CHLA to support a new foundation: CATCH! More than 400 people turned out for the inaugural picnic, including hospital staff and other volunteers.

The CATCH community now includes hundreds of children and families in Los Angeles and connects families, children, and adult mentors with children.

Events and resources for sports, music, dance, science, technology, allied mental health, psychosocial support, and prosthetics are donor supported, and CATCH has raised and distributed nearly $500,000. Over these 10 years, Dr Lightdale-Miric has seen hundreds of children with hand differences grow up and go on to medical school, performing arts programs, and collegiate sports. Together, she and the CATCH community have learned from each other and created a mission of community and a vision of meeting the individual needs of each child in the program.

Dr Lightdale-Miric's pursuit of being the best possible physician and surgeon to care for children with hand differences led her to write this book in partnership with the ASSH and AFSH as a medical voice for parents that would be distinguishable from internet information and advertising. Her goal, in her office or through this book, is to educate and empower parents of and children with hand differences to make medical decisions with up-to-date science as well as welcome a personalized approach for each individual family and child.

SARAH TUBERTY, OTD, OTR/L, grew up with a congenital limb difference. She changed schools in third grade in the middle of the 1990s with little access to images or stories of people like her. This transition was tough and really threatened her self-esteem. In the summer of 2009, Camp Winning Hands, a week-long summer camp for children 7 to 17 with congenital limb differences, began. Camp Winning Hands is hosted by the Taylor Family Foundation, UCSF Benioff Children's Hospital–Oakland, and Shriners Hospitals for Children–Northern California. Sarah has volunteered since 2009 and served on the leadership committee for several years. Each summer, parents and children expressed themselves, shared their stories, and shared their concerns, fears, and worries. Overwhelmingly, Sarah found that there was this need for content to support our parents and children with congenital limb differences.

Sarah enrolled at the Entry-Level Doctor of Occupational Therapy Program at Boston University in 2016 and graduated in 2019 with her research project being the creation of the Online Resource for Parents of Children with Congenital Hand Differences under the mentorship of her hand surgeon, Dr Michelle James. Sarah has worked to develop various resources for the disability community such as co-hosting and co-creating the *Disarming Disability Podcast* and *Super Abled Comics* and has consulted on various products, books, and media for disability representation and stigmas.

Sarah's life work is developing the resources she wished she and her parents had access to when she was younger, to help create a kinder and more inclusive world where kids feel empowered to be themselves and follow their dreams.

She presently works as a flight attendant, per diem occupational therapist at Shriners Hospitals for Children–Philadelphia, and aerial performer and adaptive circus coach with the Philadelphia School of Circus Arts. Sarah loves hikes with friends, long chats while drinking tea, and traveling the world meeting new people. She lives in the greater Philadelphia area with her partner, Erik Brewer, and their tiny jungle of house plants.

Check out more of Sarah's work at SarahTuberty.com.

References

Andersson GB, Gillberg C, Fernell E, Johansson M, Nachemson A. Children with surgically corrected hand deformities and upper limb deficiencies: self-concept and psychological well-being. *J Hand Surg Eur Vol.* 2011;36(9):795-801.

Andrews EE, Williams JL, VandeCreek L, Allen JB. Experiences of parents of children with congenital limb differences with health care providers: a qualitative study. *Rehabil Psychol.* 2009;54(2):217-221.

Ardon MS, Janssen WG, Hovius SE, Stam HJ, Selles RW. Low impact of congenital hand differences on health-related quality of life. *Arch Phys Med Rehabil.* 2015;93(2):351-357.

Bae DS, Canizares MF, Miller PE, Waters PM, Goldfarb CA. Functional impact of congenital hand differences: early results from the congenital upper limb differences (CHD) registry. *J Hand Surg Am.* 2018;43(4):321-330.

Bainbridge L. Not quite perfect! Diagnosis of a minor congenital abnormality during examination of the newborn. *Infant.* 2009;5(1):28-31.

Beresford K. Congenital hand anomaly: general considerations of care and management. *The British Journal of Hand Therapy.* 1999;4(3):112-118.

Bickham RS, Waljee JF, Chung KC, Adkinson JM. Postoperative patient- and parent-reported outcomes for children with congenital hand differences. *Plast Reconstr Surg.* 2017;139(6):1422-1429.

Birth Defects. Centers for Disease Control and Prevention. Updated October 26, 2020. Accessed December 22, 2021. https://www.cdc.gov/ncbddd/birthdefects/ul-limbreductiondefects.html.

Bond JM, Kent GG, Binney VA, Saleh M. Psychological adjustment of children awaiting limb reconstruction treatment. *Child Care Health Dev.* 1999;25(4):313-321.

Bourke G. Congenital hand anomalies. *Orthop Trauma.* 2011;25(2):143-154.

Bowen M. *Family Therapy in Clinical Practice.* Northvale, NJ: Jason Aronson, Inc, 1978.

Bradbury E. *Counseling People With Disfigurement.* Wiley-Blackwell; 1996.

Bradbury E. The psychological and social impact of disfigurement to the hand in children and adolescents. *Dev Neurorehabil.* 2007;10(2):143-148.

Brown, B. *Atlas of the Heart.* Penguin Random House LLC; 2021.

De Jong IG, Reinders-Messelink HA, Janssen WG, Poelma MJ, Van Wijk I, Van der Sluis CK. Mixed feelings of children and adolescents with unilateral congenital below elbow deficiency: an online focus group study. *PLOS ONE.* 2012;7(6)e37099.

Drotar D, Baskiewicz A, Irvin A, Kennell J, Klaus M. The adaptation of parents to the birth of an infant with a congenital malformation: a hypothetical model. *Pediatrics.* 1975;56(5):710-717.

Ezaki M. Insights into the pathogenesis of macrodactyly. *J Hand Surg Eur Vol.* 2019;44(1):25-31.

Find a Hand Surgeon. American Society for Surgery of the Hand. Updated April 2020. Accessed January 6, 2022. https://www.assh.org/handcare/fahs.

Franzblau LE, Chung KC, Carlozzi N, Chin AY, Nellans KW, Waljee JF. Coping with congenital hand differences. *Plast Reconstr Surg.* 2015;135(4):1067-1075.

Gingras G, Mongeau M, Moreault P, Dupuis M, Hebert B, Corriveau C. Congenital anomalies of the limbs: II psychological and educational aspects. *Can Med Assoc J.* 1964;91:115-119.

Goffman E. Group alignment and ego identity. In: Goffman E, ed. *Stigma: Notes on the Management of Spoiled Identity.* Prentice-Hall Inc; 1963:105-125.

Goldfarb CA, Wall LB, Bohn DC, Moen P, Van Heest AE. Epidemiology of congenital upper limb anomalies in a midwest United States population: an assessment using the Oberg, Manske, and Tonkin classification. *J Hand Surg Am.* 2015;40(1):127-132.e1-2.

Goldfarb CA, Ezaki M, Wall LB, Lam WL, Oberg KC. The Oberg-Manske-Tonkin (OMT) classification of congenital upper extremities: update for 2020. *J Hand Surg Am.* 2020;45(6):542-547.

Goodell PB, Bauer AS, Oishi S, et al. Functional assessment of children and adolescents with symbrachydactyly. *J Bone Joint Surg Am.* 2017;99(13):1119-1128.

Ho ES, Ulster AA. Evaluation of an education day for families of children with obstetrical brachial plexus palsy. *Fam Syst Health.* 2011;29(3):206-214.

Hooper B, Wood W. The philosophy of occupational therapy: a framework for practice. In: Boyt Schell BA, Gillen G, Scaffa ME, eds. Cohn E, consulting ed. *Wallard & Spackman's Occupational Therapy.* 12th ed. Lippincott Williams & Wilkins; 2014:35-45.

Huges B. Disability and the body. In: Swain J, French S, Barnes C, Thomas C, eds. *Disabling Barriers–Enabling Environments.* SAGE Publishing; 2014:55-61.

James MA, Bagley AM, Brasington K, Lutz C, McConnell S, Molitor F. Impact of prostheses on function and quality of life for children with unilateral congenital below-the-elbow deficiency. *J Bone Joint Surg.* 2006;88(11):2356-2365.

Jones NF, Kaplan J. Indications for microsurgical reconstruction of congenital hand anomalies by toe-to-hand transfers. *Hand (N Y).* 2013;8(4):367-374.

Kelley BP, Franzblau LE, Chung KC, Carlozzi N, Waljee JF. Hand function and appearance following reconstruction for congenital hand differences. *Plast Reconstr Surg.* 2016;138(1):73e-81e.

Kerr SM, McIntosh JB. Coping when a child has a disability: exploring the impact of parent-to-parent support. *Child Care Health Dev.* 2000;26(4):309-322.

Kübler-Ross E. *On Death and Dying.* Routledge; 1973.

Lightdale-Miric N, Tuberty S, Nelson D. Caring for children with congenital upper extremity differences. *J Hand Surg Am.* 2021;46(12):1105-1111.

Lumsdaine S, Thurston M. Growing up in a mainstream world: a retrospective enquiry into the childhood experiences of young adults with a physical disability. *Intl J Disabil Dev Educ.* 2016;64(2):182-197.

Mano H, Fujiwara S, Haga N. Adaptive behavior and motor skills in children with upper limb deficiency. *Prosthet Orthot Int.* 2017;42(2):236-240.

Moran SL, Jensen M, Bravo C. Amniotic band syndrome of the upper extremity: diagnosis and management. *J Am Acad Orthop Surg.* 2007;15(7):397-407.

Michielsen A, Van Wijk I, Ketelaar M. Participation and quality of life in children and adolescents with congenital limb deficiencies: a narrative review. *Prosthet Orthot Int.* 2010;34(4):351-361.

Miller CT, Kaiser CR. A theoretical perspective on coping with stigma. *J Soc Issues.* 2001;57(1):73-92.

Mpofu E. Enhancing social acceptance of early adolescents with physical disabilities: effects of role salience, peer interactions, and academic support interventions. *Intl J Disabil Dev Educ.* 2003;50(4):435-454.

Murray CE, Kelley-Soderholm EL, Murray TL. Strengths, challenges, and relational processes in families of children with congenital upper limb differences. *Fam Syst Health.* 2007;25(3):276-292.

Netscher DT, Lewis EV. Technique of nonvascularized toe phalangeal transfer and distraction lengthening in the treatment of multiple digit symbrachydactyly. *Tech Hand Up Extrem Surg.* 2008;12(2):114-120.

Occupational therapy practice framework: domain and process (3rd edition). *Am J Occup Ther.* 2014;68(suppl 1):S1-S48. doi:10.5014/ajot.2014.682006

Patterson RW, Seitz WH Jr. Nonvascularized toe phalangeal transfer and distraction lengthening for symbrachydactyly. *J Hand Surg Am.* 2010;35(4):652-658.

Pruitt S, Varni JW, Seid M, Setoguchi Y. Prosthesis satisfaction outcome measurement in pediatric limb deficiency. *Arch Physc Med Rehabil.* 1997;78:750-754.

Pruitt S, Varni JW, Seid M, Setoguchi Y. Toddlers with limb deficiency: conceptual bias and initial application of functional status outcome measure. *Arch Physc Med Rehabil.* 1999;80:819-824.

Sheffler LC, Hanley C, Bagley A, Molitor F, James MA. Comparison of self-reports and parent proxy-reports of function and quality of life of children with below-the-elbow deficiency. *J Bone Joint Surg Am.* 2009;91(12):2852-2859.

Taleporos G, McCabe M. Body image and physical disability–personal perspectives. *Soc Sci Med.* 2002;54:971-980.

Thompson A, Kent G. Adjustment to disfigurement: process involved in dealing with being visibly different. *Clin Psychol Rev.* 2001;21(5):663-682.

Tonkin MA, Oberg KC. The OMT classification of congenital anomalies of the hand and upper limb. *Hand Surg.* 2015;20(3):336-342.

Tyc V. Psychosocial adaptations of children and adolescents with limb deficiencies: a review. *Clin Psychol Rev.* 1992;12:275-291.

Wallander JL, Varni JW, Babani L, Banis HT, Wilcox KT. Family resources and resistance factors for psychological maladjustment in chronically ill and handicapped children. *J Pediatr Psychol.* 1989;14(2):157-173.

Weir S, Ephraim P, Mackenzie E. Effects of pediatric limb loss on healthcare utilization, schooling and parental labor supply. *Disabil Rehabil.* 2010;32(24):2046-2055.

Weiss A-PC, Budoff JE, Calfee RP, Goldfarb CA, Kakar S, Ladd AL, Lattanza LL, Wolf JM, eds. *The American Society for Surgery of the Hand Textbook of Hand and Upper Extremity Surgery.* 2nd ed. Chicago, IL: American Society for Surgery of the Hand; 2019.

Weiss A-PC, Goldfarb CA, Hentz VR, Raven RB III, Slutsky DJ, Steinmann SP, eds. *The American Society for Surgery of the Hand Textbook of Hand and Upper Extremity Surgery.* Chicago, IL: American Society for Surgery of the Hand; 2013.

Your Rights Under Section 504 of the Rehabilitation Act. United States Department of Health and Human Services. Updated June 2006. Accessed August 2, 2021. https://www.hhs.gov/sites/default/files/ocr/civilrights/resources/factsheets/504.pdf.

Additional Reading

For additional information, visit www.HandCare.org–a free resource from the American Society for Surgery of the Hand–where you read more on congenital hand differences and find a hand surgeon near you.

Feedback

We want your feedback!
Tell us what you thought of *The Hand Book:*